A Time
to
Care

A Time to Care

ELEANOR BLOOMFIELD

The Book Guild Ltd

First published in Great Britain in 2024 by
The Book Guild Ltd
Unit E2 Airfield Business Park,
Harrison Road, Market Harborough,
Leicestershire. LE16 7UL
Tel: 0116 2792299
www.bookguild.co.uk
Email: info@bookguild.co.uk
X: @bookguild

Typeset in 11pt Minion Pro

Printed on FSC accredited paper
Printed and bound in Great Britain by 4edge Limited

ISBN 978 1835740 569

British Library Cataloguing in Publication Data.
A catalogue record for this book is available from the British Library.

For the residents, for the staff, and for my family

CONTENTS

CONTENTS

1

COVID

Through the wall it came, a low, restless, monotonous moan, rising and falling like laboured breath: "I want to die... please let me die... I want to die... please let me die..."

I looked around for help. There was none available. Even if I pressed the staff call button, nobody would come to answer it. There were too few staff and too many people dying. It was just me and Mavis in a poky, stuffy little bedroom and an elderly lady dying on the other side of the wall.

In silence, I helped Mavis up from her wheelchair. In silence, I helped her ease creakingly onto the commode. The moans on the other side of the wall droned on. I tried to say something, anything, to drive them away, to distract Mavis, to distract myself. But my throat was dry, and no words came. I literally could not think of anything to say, mute, as in a bad dream.

Silently, I helped Mavis into her nightwear and then braced myself to help her up from the commode and onto the bed. She groaned slightly with the effort of moving but said nothing as I arranged her limbs on the mattress and pulled the thin covers up over her. When she was settled, I murmured a timid, "Goodnight," feeling the futility of the words as soon as they left my mouth. Mavis did not answer. I bent down to switch on the falls sensor beside her bed.

The tiny room was stiflingly hot. Next door the moans continued to rise and fall, holding all three of us suspended in a hellish nightmare.

I reached out a hand to open the door. Mavis had turned away from me, her face towards the wall. But she was aware of my presence, and I was still well inside the room when she suddenly burst out, pent-up fear and frustration escaping towards the wall, "Stupid woman... *shut up!*"

I was appalled, of course. But as I softly withdrew, slipping shamefully out of the room, I also silently sympathised. Mavis would get little sleep that night, doomed to lie immobile until morning, listening to Death approach on the other side of the wall.

When I left Mavis, I went and stood outside the next room, listening. I should have gone in, sat at the bedside and given what little comfort there was to give: a held hand, a smoothed forehead, a sip of water, a promise that she was not alone. But I was new and had been told that I was not to go anywhere near the 'poorlies', that only the more experienced staff – where were they? – were to deal with those patients. And so I passed quietly on down the corridor to the landing, where the evening spring light, callously beautiful, poured in through the window.

For a minute I stood there, looking with unseeing eyes at the blossom-heavy trees on the other side of the glass. Then on again down the long corridor to the door, always locked, which gave on to the staff room and the staircase beyond. One of the bedroom doors at the end of the corridor was slightly open, and from it came a tune I recognised, a violin singing high and sweet above soft massed voices: *Waltzing Matilda, waltzing Matilda, you'll come a-waltzing Matilda with me...*

I peeped in. Jack sat in the sunlight, asleep, facing a small television screen. A DVD case, *André Rieu Live in Australia*, lay beneath it.

Waltzing Matilda, waltzing Matilda...

Silently, I withdrew and pulled the door to behind me.

And his ghost may be heard as you pass by that billabong, You'll come a-waltzing Matilda with me...

I clicked the door shut and leant against it, hot tears surging up from a well of loss and grief and anger. The music played on through the closed door, carrying in its swell flooding memories of Antipodean sun, wide blue sky and rolling green seas, hitting with a force that caused actual physical pain. I looked at the threadbare carpet and chipped paint, felt the smell of bleach and death in my nostrils – no mask could keep it away – and longed desperately to be away from it all, back home, not in Australia but across the Tasman, back in New Zealand where the tui sang.

I walked on down the corridor, towards the locked door with its wire-mesh security glass.

Waltzing Matilda, waltzing Matilda, you'll come a-waltzing Matilda with me...

April 2020: one month earlier the world had turned upside down and my comfortable, privileged existence blew away

3

in the cold March wind, slipping out of reach almost before I realised it had gone. The previous December I had finished my doctorate thesis; in January I moved back to England to find work in theatre or academia. Naively, I thought there would be more opportunities in the UK, where I had been born and still held citizenship, than in the much smaller country of New Zealand. David had come out to Auckland for Christmas, and we flew back together, the plane lifting into a sky leaden with summer rain. All through November and December I had worked early and late on my thesis, racing to get it ready for submission in time for me to fly out with him. I did not want to leave home on my own, afraid that I would fail in courage and all our plans would fall apart. They did – but not in the way I, who always anticipated the worst, expected.

July was to be our wedding, in Austria, at the church where my parents and grandparents had been married before me. My wedding dress hung in my mother's wardrobe; she would bring it out with her when we met in Linz. There would be champagne and the flowers of summer, and at last I would have a photograph of my parents and all my siblings together, to frame and hang in the house we were saving hard to buy.

Auckland, Bali, Dubai, Heathrow: from summer to winter in thirty hours. England in January was miserably depressing. I slept badly, struggling with jet lag, haunted by the memory of my mother's face at the airport and of watching my father go off to work that last morning; from the dining room window I had waved to him as I always did, but I cannot remember him looking back at me, only hurrying on down the drive with head bowed.

4

But I did try, in those early, dark, cold days, to look ahead with confidence: spring would come, my thesis would return from its examination, and as soon as it did, I would be on a plane home, ready to take the viva examination and sort out my belongings to ship over to England. And once I had (hopefully) passed the viva, I could go back again, in September, to graduate. A job was so far proving frustratingly elusive, but I was steadily getting interviews; surely it was only a matter of time. We both had bad colds, but it was only a cold; it would pass. Well, yes, it *did* seem to be going on rather a long time and brought with it a horrible hacking cough that refused to shift, but perhaps we were just tired and run-down. Would I be patient, David said, I could *not* be insured on his Mini Cooper until I had learnt to drive a manual. Well, if I was that desperate to have wheels again (I was, hating and resenting the loss of freedom), here was the telephone number of the lady who had taught him and his sisters to drive. Oh, look, there were strange pictures appearing in the news coming out of China, of people in hazmat suits and having swabs stuck down their throats. Apparently, a woman in a market in Wuhan had eaten a bat and a new respiratory disease had passed from this to humans? How strange.

By early March, spring seemed as far off as ever; no word had come in relation to my thesis; all the interviews had yielded not a single job offer; and optimism – never my chief virtue – was waning fast. One freezing-cold Saturday, to quiet the raging against waste of time, money and willpower, David put me into the Mini and made me drive to Derbyshire. The car was his pride and joy, and I am still surprised he let me do this. I suppose it was a last resort, a vain hope of shutting me up. In a bitterly cold wind, we climbed Kinder Scout, and the glorious wild freedom of the Peaks was to become a solace and an escape.

On the 19th of March, Saint Joseph's feast day, we went to Mass. The church was packed, the brass on the altar gleaming gold in the candlelight. Afterwards, we went home and watched the news. We never normally did this but were vaguely alarmed by reports that something called coronavirus, or Covid, had reached the UK. Still, we were unprepared for the country being plunged into lockdown four days later.

Overnight, all my interviews were cancelled. Job listings in academia and the arts fell to nothing. Far worse, David's work – he was a self-employed dental technician, working at home with his father in a back-garden lab which blocked his mother's view from her kitchen window – came to a complete and utter stop. The lab relied on work being sent from the dentists, and the dentists were closed, along with the rest of the country. No work, no income. No money to put towards the house deposit, no money to pay the bills.

We were both living with David's parents and no future daughter-in-law was ever welcomed more warmly or more generously than I. But the entire household was dependent on the lab, and there was no furlough for the self-employed. David's wage was slashed to just enough to cover his pre-existing bills, the business bleeding capital to do even this. I, sick with worry, sat down with my laptop and looked again for work, any work.

Page after page of job listings came up. All were broadly the same, advertising for either supermarket workers or, more numerously, care workers. I sent off a flurry of applications and waited to see what would happen.

My phone rang. Could I come to an interview for the position of Care Assistant at Ember Vale Residential Care Home tomorrow morning?

I went. The home was about twenty minutes away in a part of the city I had never been to before. David drove me through streets eerily empty and waited for me in the car park.

I rang the doorbell and explained through the intercom who I was. A girl about my own age came to the door and let me in; I recognised her voice from the phone call. She showed me into a lounge adjacent to the foyer and asked me to wait.

I looked around. The room was dim and quiet. An old man sat slumped in a chair opposite me; I smiled nervously at him but was met with no response. At the other end of the room, arranged in front of windows which let in the dim spring light, a semicircle of armchairs housed more slumped figures, all apparently asleep.

A bent old lady wandered in from the foyer; she came up to me and started pulling at my hand, jabbering away in speech I could not understand. A woman wearing a green tunic hurried in behind her, stared at me with undisguised curiosity and ushered the lady away.

The girl reappeared, bearing a sheaf of papers. Would I complete these application forms? She gave me a pen, motioned towards a small table in the darkest part of the room and disappeared again.

I sat down and looked through the forms. Name, address, citizenship, did I have any criminal convictions.

Qualifications. I had none that were remotely relevant to working in care but listed my BA, then my MA, then hesitated at my PhD. I had begun my doctorate with such high hopes for the future, so many dreams of the kind of work I wanted to do: academic research, writing, dramaturgy, theatre. Those dreams had now become as fragile as gossamer, but some kind of shamed, superstitious, foolish pride held me back from putting down my doctorate, the degree I was proudest of and had been happiest completing. Sitting there that March day, I still half-believed what the prime minister had said, that the lockdown was for just three weeks while the NHS increased its capacity. Perhaps in three weeks I would be again able to apply for the jobs I had studied for, trained for, worked so hard for. Perhaps in three weeks this strange new world would be put to rights again, and no one need know that I had been forced to look for work in a care home, where I was qualified for nothing more than wiping bottoms and mopping up sick.

Experience. I had no formal experience in care but had volunteered for several years at an Auckland retirement village, working as a life story writer on a project which had initially been scheduled for six months; it had grown and expanded and was only ever finished because I had to explain that I was leaving the country. Mr Prestwick, whose memoirs I transcribed from his gentle, rambling dictation, had become a very dear friend. He enjoyed, I think, my company, and took a delightful pride in his book, which I had printed and bound for him in what was probably the university bindery's largest ever order. In turn I learnt much from him, sitting week after week in his comfortably cluttered living room, balancing alongside my laptop a cup of tea and on my knee the scone thickly spread with blackberry jam and whipped cream which he always insisted on serving me.

I had also helped care for my much-loved grandfather in the final months of his life, as he slid further and further away into dementia and physical frailty, until he no longer knew me and lay all day in the hospital bed which had been brought home for him. This had been my first sustained encounter with death, although I was not unfamiliar with it. My father worked on a neonatal intensive care unit, fighting to save tiny babies born too soon. Many survived, but many did not. As children, we were not shielded from the reality of this. Death was part of my father's job and seeped into our lives when it left him drained and exhausted, or when my mother could not hide her tears for the babies and their parents.

It wafted in, too, through the headily overpowering scent of church incense when, every year, my brothers were called on to serve the funerals of elderly members of the congregation who had been carried off by winter ailments. Sometimes I went with my mother to visit in hospital or hospice parishioners, friends, facing death, walking out of the room knowing I would never see them again except in a coffin placed feet towards the altar.

But this, living for six months with my grandparents, was the first time I had experienced the business of dying, the long, slow decline that can precede it and the way in which dementia returns the elderly to childishness again. That had been a wonderful, terrible summer, the summer of 2018 when the heat came early and blazed day after day from brilliant blue sky. I was in England for research fieldwork essential to my doctorate thesis; I worked hard, travelling thousands of miles up and down the country to libraries, archives and performances, but also enjoyed long hours and days of freedom. In the sun my hair lightened and my skin darkened; through the endless summer evenings I walked for miles over the hills or swam up and down the pool in water warm and soft as milk, watching the swallows swoop low over the house against the dusking sky. In May I met David, and summer exploded anew into fresh vitality and colour. I had never felt so alive, but all through that long season, death hovered in the midst of life.

Stonegarth had been my grandfather's home for more than fifty years. He said he would never leave it except in his coffin, and he spoke truly. But to keep him at home where he wanted to be was a huge undertaking, requiring enormous energy and sacrifice from my grandmother, whose own physical health was not the best. Carers came in once a day, then twice, then four times; a night nurse was offered but always declined. A hoist was installed in the bedroom, a chairlift fitted on the stairs. A stand-aid stood in the front hall, looking ungainly and out of place amid the antique furniture. One of the bathrooms was turned into a wet room. The care was heavy, exhausting and relentless. I helped where I could, giving meals, trying to bring him back when he wandered into the past terrors of the Finnish Winter War, staying at home to give my grandmother a few hours' respite during which she could go shopping or visit family and friends. The tension of his dying, his Finnish stubbornness carrying him on longer than the medical professionals had thought possible, became almost unbearable, until at last he slipped away just as the first faint dawn broke on another heartbreakingly fair and lovely day.

I thought of all this as I looked down at the application form, scribbled a few bare facts, then pushed the form away. The room was incredibly warm and my writing hand, clammy with heat and nerves, had left damp patches on the paper. I took off my scarf and coat. A clock on the wall ticked on into the stuffy silence.

Eventually, the girl reappeared, full of apologies for the delay, and showed me not into the manager's office but into a small room fitted out as a hair salon. Here, a few minutes later, a whirlwind appeared, pre-announced by a thunderous roll of brisk footsteps advancing down the corridor. When the dust had settled, and with it a sheaf of papers which seemed to hover like a cloud around the approaching personage, a short, brisk, sturdy woman sat in the chair opposite, legs crossed and clipboard perched atop one knee. Her face – this was still so early in the pandemic that masks had not yet appeared, not even in clinical or healthcare settings – regarded me shrewdly and keenly, but the eyes twinkled kindly, and the wide mouth was generous.

The interview was brief. I cannot now remember one word of it, but within five minutes, the whirlwind – which introduced itself as Lynn, the home manager – had uncrossed its legs, stood up, and said decidedly, "Well, Eleanor, I like you. Grace will see to your contract. When can you start?" And then, without waiting for a reply, she was gone, the thunderous footsteps hurrying off to another part of the building. On cue, Grace – who turned out to be the girl who had let me in – materialised with a brief but densely worded contract. In a daze, I signed it; still in a daze completed the next form thrust at me, which was an application for a DBS check; and still in a daze, though with a vague sense of outrage dawning, parted with £50 (non-refundable!) as application fee for said check. Grace showed me to the door and unlocked it to let me out, saying as a parting shot while punching in the numbers for the keypad: "We'll order your uniform tunic for you. It will come out of your first pay packet. Black trousers and black flat shoes your own."

The door swung shut behind me. David was waving at me from across the car park. "Well," he demanded, "how did you get on?"

"I got the job," I replied, uncertainly. I was not at all sure what I had got myself into. David was enthusiastically optimistic, but then David was always enthusiastically optimistic. I got into the car, and we drove to Sainsbury's to find black trousers and black flat shoes.

Despite the speed and alacrity with which I had got the job, it was actually nearly a month before I was able to start, because my DBS certificate took that long to come through. Grace would telephone periodically to enquire politely after its whereabouts. (At least she checked. I later learned, when it made news headlines, that other managers within the company, desperate for staff, hired new starters without undertaking the necessary DBS check. This is illegal. But so were a lot of other things that went on.) "Well," she would say, in answer to my assurance that no, I did not have it yet, "do send it through *as soon as you have it*." She always sounded faintly disbelieving, as though I were sitting on it and wickedly withholding it from her.

I both wanted, and dreaded, its arrival. I needed money. But I did not want to work in a care home.

It came on a Friday, and dutifully I emailed Grace to let her know, attaching a photograph of the certificate's front and back. My phone rang almost immediately. Could I start at 7am on Monday morning?

I seem to remember it being dark, but it was mid-April; the sky must have been lightening at least as I drove into the car park and apprehensively rang the doorbell. It pealed out shrilly through the depths of the silent building, but several minutes passed before it was opened by Lynn, preceded as before by thundering footfall. As before, she was in a hurry; she swept me up and dumped me down in the staff office, disappearing immediately on some urgent errand.

The office overflowed with lever-arch files and loose bits of paper, scattered across the desk, falling out of cupboards and drawers, spilling off shelves, even stacked in precarious piles upon the floor. One long series, housed in a big cupboard whose doors had swung open, was labelled 'care plans'; each file had a name, a number and a small photograph pasted onto the spine. Open on the desk lay a shabby red file bearing the staff rota, originally typed but with so many crossings and recrossings and handwritten amendments that it was now almost illegible. A big blue noticeboard covering most of one wall was covered with innumerable notices, all without exception bearing the words 'Covid' repeated many times over. Above the noticeboard hung a plastic clock whose hands ticked inexorably onwards towards 7am.

At 6:58am, the office began filling up with green-tunicked staff, all of whom seemingly bore large mugs of tea. One or two stared curiously, but most ignored me. All looked bone-weary, collapsing into chairs or slumping down, backs against the wall, to sit cross-legged on the floor.

The clock had ticked on to 7:04am before Lynn reappeared. "Sorry," she said briskly, "had to deal with room fourteen."

She sat down at the desk, took a piece of paper from the printer and a pen from her tunic, then pushed another piece of paper over to me. "Got a pen?"

I hadn't. She found another in the desk drawer and handed it over, then began making a list of numbers, one to thirty-nine, in two columns down the paper, motioning for me to copy her.

"Room one," she said aloud to the room in general. "Quiet night. No concerns. Room two. Fall at 12:36am. Tried to get up for the loo. Alerted by sensor. Called 999 but no visible head wound so they won't send anyone out. Said to observe. Thirty-minute obs. please for twenty-four hours. Room three. Refused personal care this morning."

And so on, up through the numbers, the staff around her scribbling brief notes and me trying to keep up. Some numbers were skipped without explanation; as my pen hovered uncertainly, the woman next to me nudged me in the ribs. "Empty," she said laconically, and showed me how on her own piece of paper she had drawn a dash against the number. Lynn was already up to number fourteen. "Passed away at 5:24am," she was saying, with no detectable change of tone. "Family told. Washed and dressed. Undertakers on the way. Let them in please when they arrive." And on their pieces of paper everyone wrote 'RIP' next to number fourteen, and the list moved on.

I remember very little of my first shifts. They passed in a hazy blur of shock. I know that by my fourth day I was working independently, completely incompetently but expected to manage because there was no other option; there were not enough staff for me to shadow for two weeks as the company handbook dictated I must. I must have been shown how to wash and dress, how to log roll a bed-bound resident to change pads or sheets or clothes, how to use the hoist and rotunda, how to answer the call bell system, how to fill in observation charts, food and fluid charts, the tick charts, the ongoing care records. But I recall nothing of this. Apart from two, I cannot even remember the deaths, although for my first six days someone new had died every time I came on shift. The two deaths I remember are the woman on the other side of the wall – but I cannot now remember her name, though straining every sinew of memory – and a man whose name, I think, was Leon. The woman through the wall haunts me still, and will forever, because I failed her so dreadfully and so completely. It was my first day, and I was alone and timid, not of Covid – which bothered me not at all, being young, fit and healthy – but of challenging orders. I should have gone in. I wish I had gone in.

In any case, the pretence of keeping new staff away from infected residents soon vanished in the wind; there were not enough staff. This was how I came to Leon on my second shift, looking down from the bedroom door as he lay on his low bed, his bare chest rising and falling with laboured breathing, his bare legs stick-thin. He had 'crashed' – deteriorated suddenly and rapidly – and the ambulance staff had been called out. I had been sent to see if they needed anything. Many paramedics were very good, kind and assured with the residents, able to share a joke with the staff. But some hated being sent to the care homes, could not wait to leave, and – resplendent in their gold-crested uniforms and smug in their NHS status – looked down on the care staff as inferior beings. These paramedics were of the latter kind. Leon's temperature had soared to 39.9°C – he was sweating profusely and burning hot to the touch – this was why, in an attempt to make him more comfortable, his outer clothes and the top bedding had been removed. But the paramedics sniffily said this was undignified and sent me to get a sheet 'to cover him up'. Down I meekly trotted to look for one in the laundry. I got back slightly out of breath, having had to search the whole building for a clean, dry, ironed sheet, just as they were transferring Leon – none too gently – onto the ambulance stretcher. The nearest paramedic took the proffered sheet without a word of thanks or acknowledgement. And, shrouded in my sheet, Leon was carted off to hospital, and by the next shift, he was dead, and we never saw him again.

A few other memories remain, brief moments of lucidity in a jumbled and garish nightmare.

Trying to help residents talk to their families. Both the Wi-Fi and phone signal barely reached beyond the staff office, which meant that in the bedrooms – to which the residents were confined for weeks – telephone calls and Facetime videos were always cutting out, if they ever connected in the first place. Giving up and going back to the office, there to tell a frantic relative that Mum was OK, yes really, yes we would let them know if there was any change, no we didn't know when visiting would be allowed again, don't worry, we will look after Mum, she's getting the best of care. Learning to lie.

Clanging the meal trolleys up and down the corridors, delivering dinners to each isolated inmate in their cell. The noise of the ancient, unwieldy trolleys, rattling with crockery and cutlery, was – almost literally – enough to wake the dead.

Kitty, who would not stay in her room, shuffling endlessly up and down the corridor, calling for her twin. She was classed as a high falls risk and a motion sensor was set up in her bedroom to detect whenever she moved from her chair. It was continually, everlastingly going off, and we were continually, everlastingly, ushering Kitty back to her room.

Chelsea – exhausted after working fourteen days in a row, hounded by the endless high-pitched beeping of the call bells and sensors – snapping on her fourteenth back-to-back twelve-hour shift, snarling at everyone and no one, "Shut up, *shut the fuck up!*"

Most farcical of all, in the endless saga of ever-changing Covid policies and procedures, there was the Episode of the Michelin Man Painting Suits. Apart from one day when we ran out of masks, there was never, at Ember Vale, the shortage of PPE that was reported at some other care homes. But the company director woke up one morning and decided, motivated not out of concern for his staff but out of concern for his public image, that double gloves, double masks, double aprons, shoe protectors, goggles and visors were insufficient, and staff working with Covid-positive residents should have Extra Protection. And this Extra Protection? Lynn was sent out to Wilko to buy three sets of overalls – the disposable kind, made out of a kind of fabric paper, that you use to protect hair and clothes from home DIY. They cost about £2. These were presented to us at the morning handover, and we were informed that those of us looking after the 'poorlies', as the Covid patients were euphemistically termed, had to wear them.

Care homes in lockdown were not repositories of practical jokes. Nevertheless, we enquired blankly if this was one.

No, we had to wear them. Hood up and all.

We struggled into them in the toilets and, clumsy in the confined space, I caught my heel in one of the trouser legs. The flimsy fabric tore immediately. Oops.

Over the top went the double aprons and the shoe protectors. I was sweating even before emerging from the toilets. Care work is hard, physical and hurried, and in the sultry artificial heat, all the suits were, by the mid-morning break, fetid. Designed, presumably, for men, they were far too big for most of us and, as we rushed up and down the corridors, billowed out around our perspiring forms like an inflating tyre. For one day only, sweating, cursing, green-tunicked carers were replaced by sweating, cursing Michelin Men.

In the evening, at the end of the shift, gloves, aprons, masks and shoe protectors went in the yellow clinical waste bins; goggles and visors went in buckets of disinfectant; and we were told to hand over the painting suits – torn, ragged, dirty and smelly – to the night staff. Straight away. No, there was no time to wash them. No, there weren't any fresh suits. Three was all we had, and we had to reuse them.

There was a riot.

Perhaps wisely, Lynn had already left for the night. Definitely wisely, the painting suits were quietly allowed to disappear. There was no trace of them the next morning, and they were never mentioned again.

The only part of my uniform I still have is the fob watch. When I eventually realised that I was finally free of Ember Vale, I promptly threw out everything else in a cathartic purge – green tunic, black trousers, black shoes, name badge, all the endless hateful blue masks knocking around unhygienically at the bottom of my work bag, even the bag itself. (I really wanted to burn them, but it was early spring, and I had just reseeded my lawn.) I don't know why I kept the watch; I will, hopefully, never wear it again. It was a little metal nurse's fob watch, the kind that pins on the breast of your uniform and hangs there upside down, so that when you look down at it, the time stares back at you right way up. It was a cheap little thing, bought from some now-forgotten online shop, but it lasted my time at Ember Vale. The battery has run down now, the comforting tiny tick of the second hand dead. But I still have it.

People often speak, now, of the 'lost years' of the lockdowns and restrictions. For many it seems that life stopped at the end of 2019 and is only just now beginning to re-establish itself. While everyone else had too much time those long summer months of 2020, in care work there is never, ever enough. With time pinned onto the front of our tunics, we were always trying to outrun the second hand, keep up with the relentless march of the minute hand. In a care home, time is both acutely observed and intensely meaningless. You are always aware of the clock, trying to squeeze an impossible number of tasks into an impossibly short time frame, forever documenting time and date on care records and observation charts and incident forms. And yet it is all pointless, for all the same tasks will have to be done all over again the next day, at the same time, with the same lack of time, and every day is the same as the days preceding and the days following, and never more so than in lockdown.

I genuinely cannot remember how long the home operated under the warped timing of its harshest lockdown, when all the residents were confined to their own tiny rooms and the shift schedule operated on a day and night pattern, twelve hours each, rather than the usual triad of morning, afternoon and night. But it was too long for those residents who, by the time they were allowed out again, had forgotten how to wash, dress and feed themselves, use a toilet, recognise family and friends, even to speak. Normality – or what passes for normality in residential care – still had not returned to the home when I left it two years later.

Lockdowns, we all hope, are a thing firmly of the past. Looking back, they seem vague and unreal sometimes now, like a confused dream where nothing makes sense. Did we really follow all those silly rules, while politicians partied and people in care homes, nursing homes, hospitals, died alone and friendless? Did we really obey so blindly, care so little?

Time has passed since I worked at Ember Vale and much has changed; my life now is very different, much more secure (although is anything ever really secure?), much happier. And yet for me the care home is not a thing of the past. Sometimes I forget it in the busyness of life, but then I will meet a sight, a sound, a smell, and be instantly transported back, back to misery and despair and death. Time has not dulled Ember Vale. Instead, I have become slightly obsessed with time, fascinated with the way it can hang so heavy or slip away like grains of sand falling through cupped fingers. I wonder at the way it collapses under the pressure of dementia, so that my grandmother can ask me in one breath how my babies are, and in the next worry that she has not recently called her parents, dead for forty years. In the world, in life, we never have enough time. Residents of care homes have too much time. There is a lesson here somewhere, but I'm not sure what it is. I only remember Angela, late one Sunday evening, resisting her weekly shower. One after another we tried to coax her into the bathroom, until it was my turn.

"You stupid woman!" she snapped (all of the carers were stupid women). "I haven't got time for this! I've got to put the horses to bed!" *Oh, Angela,* I thought sadly, *you have all the time in the world, for all the good it may do you, for you will never put the horses to bed again.*

They say – that old cliché – that what doesn't kill you makes you stronger. Working in a care home did not kill me, but I do not feel, yet, that it made me stronger. It pushed me towards an abyss on whose edge I still wobble and teeter. The pandemic hardened all my pre-existing faults and brought out into even sharper relief the negative aspects of my personality. Patience has completely deserted me. David, the most easy-going person I have ever met, now becomes impatient at my impatience, while his boundless optimism – the reason I married him! – I often resent. More than ever, I expect the worst to happen, and when it doesn't, I am mistrustful: it must be a trick, disaster has been merely diverted, not avoided. I worry far too much about whether the bills for the month are covered. The thought of the lab being again unable to support us, now that we have a mortgage and two small children, terrifies me even more than it did four years ago. I miss my family with a terrible aching fear that I will again be shut out of my country, unable to get back to them if I need to. And the care home haunts my dreams, still and forever. I left, but it will not leave me.

2

HOME SWEET HOME

A care home is, unpleasantly, a type of prison. It is designed to be difficult to get into, and even harder to get out of. External doors are kept permanently locked, secured with keypads or alarms or both. Internal doors connecting different parts of the building are also always locked. Windows are fixed to open only a crack. Some homes have CCTV cameras trained on the communal areas. However appealing the surface gilt – the fresh paint, the fresh flowers, the scented incense sticks, the photograph board of smiling staff – the unappealing reality is, ultimately, impossible to disguise.

Ember Vale Residential Care Home made no pretence whatsoever of possessing even the thinnest layer of surface gilt. It was – is – a thoroughly ugly and thoroughly depressing 1960s building of dark grey brick. Built to be grimly functional, it made not the slightest attempt at aesthetic appeal. The building felt run-down and unloved, although it was not uncared for. The paintwork was relatively new; manager and staff made valiant attempts to brighten the interior with artwork and cheery placards. The latter were of the kind that say *Home Is Where the Heart Is* and *Follow Your Dreams* and *Live, Love, Laugh*; in such a setting, at such a time, they seemed supremely incongruous and vaguely inappropriate. The foyer was always decorated for holidays or according to the seasons; after Halloween there was a glut of pumpkins, which the residents ate for days as soup, and one of them came home with me to be turned into a jack-o'-lantern. A few rose bushes struggled bravely at the front; one of them had for a few weeks of the year gorgeous heavy yellow blooms, but somehow they were overpowered and tainted by the dull grey wall behind. Normally, I cannot walk past a rose bush in bloom without itching to pluck its flowers to adorn my bedroom, but those roses survived unscathed for two long summers.

There was a small garden, which, because it was enclosed, I called a courtyard garden, earning for this some ridicule and accusations of being 'posh'. Three sides were formed by the arms of the building and the fourth by a high wood and wire fence that would not have looked out of place in Stalag Luft III. Apart from this, the garden was the most pleasant place in the entire home. When the weather was warm enough, I always took my breaks there instead of in the tiny, smelly staff room. A tall slender birch tree grew out of the grass, and I would sit at the base of this with my back against the trunk, looking up at the green leaves against blue sky and willing to escape. If the ground was wet, I perched on one of the wooden benches, whose end was overgrown by tall rushes; into these I would press myself, trying to disappear and hoping that no one could find me.

In normal times, the garden was cared for by the daughter of one of the residents. With lockdown it became wild and overgrown, but in summer I used to pick little posies of whatever flowers and greenery still flourished and take them home with me to decorate my bedside table. I tried to do this stealthily, feeling rather guilty, but when eventually I was spotted, other people started doing the same, and for the brief time of high summer, staff would leave through the front door at the end of shifts clutching disposable plastic drinking cups stuffed full of half-wilting flowers.

Ember Vale had rooms for thirty-nine residents, making it a mid-size home. The odd number of rooms puzzled me until I learnt that originally, there had been thirty-eight; one day the owner decided to take the staff room and the kitchen used by the residents' families and make it thirty-nine. More rooms, more money. Most of the bedrooms were tiny. If the occupant was fully mobile, this was manageable, just, but more often the resident, a wheelchair, two carers and the hoist or rotunda would all be tangled up together, struggling to manoeuvre in a room about three metres by two. Most of the space was taken up by the bed; these were all hospital beds – visually unappealing but surprisingly comfortable, as I found when I spent a night in one on call. Each room also had a wardrobe, a sink with a mirror above and built-in cupboard below, and an armchair. That was all, except for six rooms at the ends of the wings: these were slightly larger, with space for two armchairs instead of one, or a small chest of drawers in addition to the wardrobe. Only two rooms out of the thirty-nine had an en-suite toilet and shower.

During the first lockdown, each resident was 'requested' to remain in isolation in their own room. This incarceration – there really is no other word for it – went on for weeks. The bedroom doors, all gaily painted in different bright colours, were not locked; not even in the name of Covid did infection control policy dare to go quite that far. But 'wanderers' had the door alarms on their rooms activated, and if any resident so much as poked their nose out of their door, a member of staff swooped down and shooed them back inside. The two residents with en-suite toilets were lucky; everyone else had to make do with commodes.

There was a large dining room and five assorted lounges of different sizes. One of these opened into a conservatory, which in warm weather became so unbearably hot that it had to be taken out of use; the fan was broken and several of the windows could not be opened. There were several mixed-sex toilets and three wet rooms; there was also a bath, which I never saw used; the room was used instead to store equipment and continence aids. At the end of one wing was the laundry, to which I was always glad to escape for a minute or two while searching for clean sheets or clean knickers, which were in eternally short supply. The noise of the big machines drowned out the ever-present ringing of the bells, and there was always a warm welcome from the two laundry assistants, who, taking pity on us, would welcome us into a haven of comparative peace.

The two floors of the building were connected by three staircases at the ends of the corridors and, right in the middle of the building, one antiquated, hated lift. In the whole time I was at Ember Vale, it never worked properly. The doors, instead of closing smoothly, juddered and jerked, opened again, stuttered back towards the middle, stuck fast, then decided to open again and remain open. Often you had to physically force them closed in order to set the lift in motion. If you did manage to complete a journey and emerge, giving thanks that you had survived one more trip in the Beast, you had to remember to close the doors behind you after exiting. If you did not, they remained open and the lift remained where it was so that if you were on the other level, it could not be called down. When this happened to you, you stood, cursing, with a finger on the button; this then emitted a furious buzzing which you hoped would be heard by someone working on the other level and correctly interpreted as a signal to close the doors. But if nobody heard, you had to go back along the corridor and up the stairs, back again along the corridor to descend in the lift (cursing of course at the doors as they struggled to close), pick up your wheelchair passenger from below and ascend again with yet more curses.

Once a month or so, the lift would pack up completely. A notice would go up on the doors – *Lift out of order* – we would groan and swear at the added difficulty this created in an already overstretched shift, and an engineer would appear to fiddle around in the lift well. Whatever he did never worked. After a couple of hours he would disappear, the lift would be back in use with no discernible difference, and a few weeks later, it would happen all over again. The solution, of course, would have been to install a new lift, but that meant spending money. So it was never fixed and we struggled on.

Stationed at various points along the corridors were the dashboards to which the call bell system was connected. These were always positioned in the most inconvenient places, so that you had to go along the corridor to see who was ringing, and then back again to answer it. There was no dashboard in, or even near, the biggest lounge; if it was noisy in there, you could not hear the bells at all, and then you would be yelled at for failing to answer them.

Beneath the bright paint, the building was run-down. There was the lift, and the broken fan in the conservatory, and towards the end of my time working there, the call bell system started playing up. The lights in the corridors were faulty and electricians appeared with about the same regularity as the lift engineer. They would stand on ladders in the middle of the corridors with their heads up inside a hole they had made in the ceiling, subjecting the wiring to mysterious operations that never seemed to make any appreciable difference to the lighting. The corridors were not wide enough for us to pass with wheelchairs, so every time we went by with one, the electricians had to climb down from their ladder, move it to the side, wait for us to pass, then put the ladder back and ascend again.

Things were never fixed – or, if they were, like the lighting and the lift, never done properly. The equipment – hoists and rotundas – was old and ungainly, heavy to push and hard to manoeuvre. The batteries on the hoists were faulty and frequently the machinery refused to operate even with a fresh one fitted. The two hoists, one on each floor, took it in turns to break more completely and be taken away for servicing. With one hoist out of action, the time pressures of care, already insane, grew even more ridiculous. One of the residents had paid for a ceiling hoist to be fitted in her bedroom, which would have made life easier both for her and us, but it had broken long before I arrived, and broken it remained.

One day shortly after Christmas, the morning shift came on to find no hot water anywhere in the building. Bedrooms, bathrooms, kitchen, laundry: all ran cold. Showering anybody was obviously out of the question. Nevertheless, it was equally out of the question that people be got up without some kind of wash. It was midwinter, and using cold tap water was impossible. We ended up filling the tea jugs with boiling water from the kitchen urn and staggering upstairs with them like Victorian housemaids, having to mix the water to the right temperature with the cold water in the washbasins. Of course, this took extra time; of course, people were late getting up; of course, the senior wanted to know why.

By lunchtime, the hot water had reappeared, but the next morning it was again running cold. I told Lynn, hurrying by on her way to interview yet another potential new staff member over WhatsApp. (Mine was the last in-person interview ever held for the duration of the pandemic. After that, as an infection control procedure, they were held over video call.)

"It was fixed yesterday," she said.

"Well, it's off again now," I said.

She insisted it was fixed. I insisted it was cold. The stand-off was only brought to an end by another carer coming to report that parts of the building appeared to have hot water but not others. So we had to go through the bedrooms one by one, running the taps to find out which had hot water and which didn't, and making a list of the affected rooms for Lynn to hand on to the plumbers (who insisted that they had fixed the entire building the previous day). More time wasted, late again getting people up, another senior demanding to know why the dining room was not cleared by 9:30am.

The entire home was incredibly warm. This was pleasant if it was snowing outside, and extremely unpleasant the rest of the time. Yes, the elderly feel the cold, but that doesn't mean that they wish to be broiled alive. The heating system, like the rest of the building, was antiquated; whatever the outside temperature, it could not be switched off or even turned down. A few of the radiators could be turned off individually, but most of them simply blasted out unremitting heat twenty-four hours a day. As the windows only opened to a gap of a few centimetres, there was no way of cooling the air temperature. Some of the residents, stewing in chairs all day beside the hard-working radiators, found the dry, stuffy heat acutely distressing. But there was nothing we could do apart from remove outer layers of clothing, attempt to move them out of the sunlight or proffer sips of water in flimsy plastic cups.

In summer, the heat was appalling. As the outside temperatures climbed through the twenties and even into the thirties, hot sun blazing down from cloudless blue sky, the radiators remained on. Pushing a wheelchair down the corridor was enough to break perspiration. Putting someone to bed would leave us pouring with sweat, tunics sticking damply to puffing torsos. There was a constant stream of staff through the kitchen to the cold tap, where we fought over the limited supply of glasses, filling them again and again, downing a pint at a time. It was impossible to work quickly; the oppressive heat sapped energy, leaving everyone in the building lethargic and exhausted. And management wondered why so many of the residents showed signs of dehydration!

By the second summer, I was nearly twenty-eight weeks pregnant, and it occurs to me now, looking back, that working in such conditions was frankly dangerous. The staff room, no doubt in a nod towards employees' rights to tolerable working conditions, had an ancient air conditioning unit mounted on one wall. However, this nod was more of a slap in the face, for the air conditioning made no appreciable difference to the temperature, was so loud when in operation that it was impossible to hold a conversation, and stank. In hot weather, more of the staff took to joining me in spending their breaks outside, and at the end of shifts, we would all crowd onto the patio area in search of cooler air in which to complete our paperwork.

The unyielding heat remains something of a mystery to me, for running it at perpetual full tilt must have added hugely to the home's running costs and cut heavily into the all-important profit margins. I can only conclude that either the cost of upgrading the system was more than the owner was willing to pay or that it was an insurance policy against possible accusations of not keeping the elderly warm enough. So staff and residents sweltered together in misery.

The warmth of the building, and the lack of fresh air, contributed to the smell. No amount of bleach or air freshener, squirted liberally each shift by the domestic staff, ever quite succeeded in masking this. It lingered in the corridors, pervading the curtains, carpets and upholstery: the smell of quiet despair. Not quite definable but instantly recognisable, it was the stale smell of unhappy old age: urine and shit and blood and sweat and old food and mustiness and misery and lack of hope. The domestics scrubbed daily, but the smell always won. We carried it around with us as we worked and home again at the end of each shift. It clung to hair and clothing, so pervasively that the only way to be rid of it was with a hot wash. Not only our uniforms smelt, but our ordinary clothes as well, even though we changed out of them before every shift; into the wash they went before I could bear to wear them again. I always walked out feeling disgustingly dirty, heading for the shower as soon as I got home. I disliked hugging David before washing, worried not only that he would be repelled but that the smell would taint him too. The throes of working through morning sickness were made worse by becoming simply too sick and too tired to shower after getting home; I would collapse into bed, dirty and miserable, still smelling the care home and hearing its bells, never able to escape.

Never forget, we were exhorted regularly in staff meetings and by notices pinned up in office and staff room, *that this may be your place of work, but it is also our residents' home.*

This was simply untrue. The care home might have been where they lived, but it was not 'home' to its residents, most of whom – as Lynn freely admitted one staff meeting – were there against their will. How could it be, with its bells and sensors and sterility and tiny bare rooms and shared bathrooms and lack of privacy and institutionalised routine – how could this ever be 'home'? How could anyone ever pretend that it was?

A scene one morning with Marion only emphasised this. Marion had a reputation as 'difficult', which she had earned five minutes after entering the care home. Vicious and vindictive, she was outrageously rude to staff and caused trouble among the other residents. Nobody liked dealing with her, and she was avoided wherever possible. This was easy, because she still had full capacity and was still entirely independent; in fact, she should not have been in a residential care home at all. It was ill-suited to her needs, and she had clearly not settled there.

This particular morning, I passed her room, hurrying down the corridor on some now-forgotten errand. Raised angry voices floated out from beneath Marion's closed bedroom door. I hesitated. I had no time and no desire to get involved. But...

I knocked and peered round the door. Before I could enquire, another carer shot out and disappeared down the corridor, only too glad to make her escape. I was left with an extremely irate elderly lady ranting that the staff were rude (rich!), that her bed had not been made satisfactorily (this was because she was sitting on it), that her morning tea had been cold (probably true), that her underwear had been lost in the wash (more than likely) and that, in general, the service was unacceptable (fair, but not our fault). I attempted to break into this flow, but she rounded on me, threatening to report me (what for was not clear, but I did not doubt that she was capable of inventing something) and have me sacked.

I shut up. Whatever I said was clearly only going to make matters worse, yet I could not walk away; she was in a state close to hysteria. Not knowing what else to do, I sat down on the bed beside her and waited for the storm to abate.

The storm did not abate, but its focus shifted. Out spilled misery and frustration, anger and pure anguish. Not really talking to me, but needing someone to listen, she began to explain how her husband had died a few months before, how her children had told her she could no longer manage on her own, how her home had been sold by them against her will (perhaps unwisely, she had apparently given them power of attorney). How she had been packed off to the care home with only a few days' notice. How she both hated her children for what they had done and missed them dreadfully. How wrong it was that she could see them only through a closed window for a few minutes at a time. How her once-prized possessions had been reduced to a few clothes and a couple of knick-knacks. And how she missed her two cats.

With the cats a torrent of tears was finally unleashed. Grief rolled out, raw and devastating, but no longer hysterical. I took her hand, and she did not push me away.

She had not been allowed to bring the cats with her into the care home and did not know what had happened to them; her children would not tell her. She suspected, probably with good reason, that her cherished pets had simply been put down.

I did not really like Marion any better after this episode, but I understood her better and had far more sympathy for her. It was obvious that most of her difficult behaviour sprang from the fact that she was desperately unhappy, and for this I could not blame her. In the same situation, I am sure I would behave no better.

I could not understand her children, nor the reason for their cruelty and their betrayal. Sadly, though, Marion's was a story we saw repeated again and again; it was, in fact, the normal story behind most of the new admissions. *You can't manage on your own anymore*, families say, *off you go to a care home*. Marion should have been supported to remain in her own home for as long as possible, since those were clearly her wishes and she was not in any way incapacitated. Instead, she was made wretchedly, needlessly miserable, losing at a stroke her home, her possessions, her independence, her pride and her beloved cats.

Marion never settled at Ember Vale, continuing to create discord among both staff and residents. It ended when she verbally threatened another resident; the police were called in, much to the indignation of her children, who then laid a complaint against the care home. It had no possible basis and was easily dealt with. But Marion's position in the home had clearly become untenable, and one day she was gone.

And that was that. Except that it wasn't. Marion haunts me to this day. Haunting me even more are the lost ghosts, those whose dementia meant they were quite incapable of grasping the permanent change in their surroundings or the reason for it. So many times an anxious, questing face would be upturned to mine, and a quavering voice would ask, "When am I going home?" Julian used to pack his suitcase, over and over again, and politely ask us to call a taxi: "Because it's time I went home now." I hated having to say, as gently as possible, "This is your home now; this is where you live." But the lie of "It's just for tonight, we'll take you home in the morning," was the one lie I could never bring myself to tell.

I was something of a lost ghost myself when I started working at Ember Vale, not quite sure where I belonged. What I still considered my home was twelve thousand miles away in New Zealand. I had left this home with all kinds of plans for the future, plans which were ground down by a grey English winter and then completely obliterated by the lockdown. Although I had known leaving home would be difficult, I was utterly unprepared for an enforced exile. I left in January thinking I would be back in May to sit my PhD viva. Instead, it would be more than two years before the New Zealand border reopened, and I still have not returned. Underlying the ache for home is a terrible sense of guilt; I simply flew away from my family one day and never came back. I left so many things unfinished, and now I cannot get back.

One freezing cold day early in 2020, just before Covid crashed into the UK, David and I went to the bank to see about getting a mortgage; we would need somewhere to live after the wedding, and neither of us wanted to rent. The outcome of the meeting was not encouraging. Unemployed, I was classed as dependent on him (how this stung). With this encumbrance, and on David's income alone, there was no way we could afford to buy anything. Clearly, I needed to find work as soon as possible. Then along came the lockdowns.

A home of our own became as remote a possibility as getting to Mars. Luckily for us, David's parents could not have been kinder or more generous. They had taken me in when we arrived back from New Zealand, and it would be more than a year before they finally got rid of us (and all the stuff we had accumulated, which entirely filled their front room). A year after I went for the interview at Ember Vale we had, against all the odds, somehow succeeded in buying our own home. Much as I hated working at the care home, it was this job that secured our house.

By a quirk of urban layout, moving house did not alter my journey time to work. I used to time this by Classic FM; if the 6:30am news came on before I reached the Brownhill Roundabout, then I was running late for the morning shift. At lunchtime, heading in for the afternoon shift, the journey always took longer, the time gradually creeping up as the lockdowns eased; eventually, I had to start leaving earlier and earlier to allow for the traffic. But in all the time I worked there, I was never late, although the senior frowned at me when I once – only once! – walked through the door at precisely 2pm. Coming home at night, with clear roads and green lights, I used to race back as quickly as possible. Night after night, speeding through the dark, I would have one eye on the clock, trying to beat previous records. The quickest I ever managed was seventeen minutes; during the day, the same journey could sometimes take forty minutes or more.

Somehow, I never got a speeding ticket. I knew where the cameras were and how to avoid them, although I was lucky never to get caught by a mobile patrol. I never drove recklessly, but I was always desperate to get away, to put as much space as possible between myself and the shift, to get into another space where I could breathe freely and attempt to forget about work. I knew the roads and the traffic light timings so well that, if David ever picked me up and drove home, I would berate him for his slower progress. "Hurry up," I would say, "if you put your foot down now you'll get through that light." Or, on a forty-mile-an-hour road, "You can do forty-seven down here – the speedo reads fast." I think he thought I was joking, but I wasn't. I wasn't quite sure where home was, but it sure as hell wasn't the care home.

"You'd better take that off," Sheryl said. "NG's here."

I looked down at my engagement ring. At first, I took it off for work, but since the cancellation of our wedding, I had become reluctant to remove it. I suppose I wore it as a token, a symbol that one day things would improve, and plans unmade would come again to fruition. But the uniform policy stated that one could wear only a wedding ring. Sheryl knew, and I knew, that if NG saw me wearing it, he would be within his rights to sack me. And although he didn't care two straws for the rights of his employees, he would not hesitate to exercise his own. I took off the ring and slipped it into the pen pocket of my tunic.

NG – who shall remain nameless, not that he deserves it – was always referred to among the staff by his initials. He was the owner of the home and soundly despised by every single member of staff below Lynn. Lynn was far too discreet to share publicly in the disdain expressed by the rest of the staff but made little attempt to contain it.

Around 84% of care home beds in England today are provided by private companies. NG headed two of these. The homes were, of course, run for profit; I do not believe NG had an ounce of care or compassion in his entire body. He treated his staff appallingly, viewing them as merely expendable commodities. At the time I joined the company he was engaged in overhauling the staff contracts, aggressively cutting pay and informing anyone resisting that they would lose their job. In fact, we were always being threatened with losing our jobs, for anything from smoking on site to failing to wear PPE correctly. Emails reminding us of these transgressions, and the fact that they constituted GROSS MISCONDUCT – he was fond of capitals – would appear regularly on the staff room noticeboard, and we would all be expected to sign beneath his hated name to say that we had 'read and acknowledged'.

The scandal over contracts made the local media. So did the fact that one of Ember Vale's sister homes suffered emergency closure, having spectacularly failed an inspection. The company was still left, however, with twelve homes, of which one third received a 'requires improvement' rating in 2021. According to staff who had worked across different homes, Ember Vale was one of the nice ones. We were all forbidden, of course, to talk to the media. NG, adopting a tone shocked and sorrowful, attempted to frame the negative press as the malicious gossip of one or two wicked members of staff. But the media didn't know the half of it.

About once a month or so, NG would appear in person, to prowl around the home and then sit closeted in Lynn's office while the kitchen staff provided him with tea, served in the best china which never normally made an appearance. He would arrive unannounced in his big fancy car, behind whose tinted windows he once waited in order to catch Leila in the act of smoking a forbidden cigarette outside the kitchen door. He actually took a photograph of her doing so and then leapt into the home brandishing his phone and raising hell with Lynn for allowing the staff to smoke on site. Leila thought her time was up, but of course he couldn't actually sack her, for it would have left the home even more chronically understaffed than it already was. He simply liked to intimidate and to humiliate; he was, in short, an arrogant bully.

Short and rotund, he strutted around like a sleek fat cat. He always wore a dark grey suit and gold-rimmed glasses, oozing ostentation and money from every pore. He had peculiar obsessions; we all had to wear black ballerina-type pumps rather than any other kind of footwear (these are bad for the feet, offering no support for the arch and no protection for the toes against mis-steered wheelchairs or roving equipment). One day he suddenly decreed that all the sandwiches served for tea should have their crusts cut off, because that was how he liked his own sandwiches. The kitchen staff disliked the extra work and the residents complained; the sandwiches were about half the size they had been and, with no crusts to hold them together, fell apart. Not even NG could pretend that his own sandwich preferences should override the residents', but, in order to save face, half the sandwiches were then served without crusts while the other half was permitted to retain theirs.

A good employer learns his employees' names, speaks to them when he encounters them, attempts to discover if they are happy in their work. NG did none of these things. He treated all his staff as beneath contempt and inevitably was heartily detested in return. Whenever he was on the prowl, we all tried to keep well out of the way. Running into each other, we would anxiously ask, "Is he still here?" and when finally the big car drove off up the drive, everyone breathed a collective sigh of relief. I only ever spoke one word to him, one day when my preferred tactic for hiding somewhere at the back of the building went awry. Coming hurriedly through a door, I met him on the other side, nearly bumping into him in my haste. He stood there, pompous as ever, looking for all the world as if he expected me to curtsey to him. Well, *kiss my arse*, I thought, and waited to see what would happen. I was taller than him and took considerable satisfaction, as well as courage, from this. A few seconds passed. Then: "Hello," he said. "Hello," I said politely and waited again. But he said nothing more, simply passed me by and carried on down the corridor.

Early in 2021, a rumour started, and soon spread around the staff like wildfire, to the effect that NG had himself been diagnosed with early onset dementia and that his son would be taking over the company. Morality deserting me, I could not help but consider this poetic justice. And if he ends up in one of his own care homes, well, that would be revenge sweet indeed.

3

RESIDENTS

"I don't know where I am," quavered the old, broken voice. "Where am I?"

"At Ember Vale Care Home," I answered automatically, scribbling furiously to get my paperwork done within the last ten minutes of the shift.

"I don't know what I'm doing," the plaintive voice continued.

"You're just sitting relaxing in the lounge," I replied, trying to sound calm and soothing while writing that the resident whose care record I was updating had that morning scratched, hit and bitten me before unleashing a string of quite impressively bad words.

"I don't know what I'm doing," the voice repeated again, rising quickly into a piercing shriek. "Help! Help! Help!"

I jumped up, scattering papers and files across the table.

"Simone! It's all right! Shush, don't shout. Everything's fine, look, you're at home, in the lounge. Look, I'll get you a nice cup of tea."

Cries of "Help! Help!" pursued me into the kitchen. By the time I got back three minutes later with the tea, it was to a scene of uproar. Simone was still screaming; two other carers were trying without success to reassure her; and Cindy was wheeling herself about in her wheelchair demanding that 'that woman' should 'shut up'. I removed Cindy as far as possible from the melee and tried, unsuccessfully, to distract Simone with the tea. She pushed me away, causing pale, lukewarm tea – we were taught to make it horribly milky so that it did not scald when, inevitably, it spilled – to cascade down my tunic and onto the floor. Off I went to get mop and sponge and the obligatory *Wet floor* sign. All the while, Simone continued screaming, and as I fled through the front door at the end of the shift, the screams pursued me still.

Dementia is a terrible condition, one I would not wish on anyone. No – not even, really, on NG. As people continue to live longer, and other physical conditions become increasingly treatable, it is also becoming more and more common. If nothing else gets you in the end, then the likelihood is dementia will. It is more common in women than men, in part because women tend to live longer. Around 850,000 people in the UK are currently living with dementia, a figure the NHS estimates will rise to more than one million by 2025. In terms of population, this is about one in forty, the same as the number of staff working for the NHS, whose website points out that this figure means you probably know at least one NHS staff member. By the same logic this means that most people will, at some point, experience the ravages of dementia – if not suffering from it themselves then by proxy, watching a loved one fall prey to its clutches.

There are various forms of dementia. Alzheimer's is the most common of these, but there is also a wider array, including vascular dementia, Lewy body dementia, frontotemporal dementia and dementia associated with Parkinson's disease. There is currently no cure and no treatments that can address the underlying cause rather than the symptoms. The most common effect – the symptom most patients first present with, and the one that springs immediately to mind whenever anyone says the word *dementia* – is memory loss, specifically loss of short-term memories and the inability to form new ones. It begins insidiously, what used to be called the 'benign forgetfulness of old age' – misplacing your glasses or keys, perhaps repeating yourself a bit in conversation – but as it advances, there is nothing remotely benign about it, although not everyone reaches its final stages. To me, the two saddest things to witness are sufferers asking where their dead spouse is, forgetting that they died long ago, and the terrible point when they no longer recognise their own friends and family.

As dementia advances, many people – especially if they are shut away from family and stimulation – withdraw from the present and seek refuge in the past, reliving events that took place in childhood or young adulthood. Sometimes these memories are traumatic. I can still hear my grandfather shouting out in Swedish, "The Russians are coming! The Russians are coming!", his wide eyes seeing not our cosy television room but the invasion of Finland in the Winter War. He would have been about twelve at the time. I barely understood the words – an uncle translated them – but their fear and urgency still causes me to shiver. And I still mourn the fact that, no matter how hard we tried, we could not recall him to the safety of the present, only watch and wait and hope his mind would eventually let him back. Sometimes, though, the past can be safer than the present. If someone is convinced their spouse is still alive, trying to convince them otherwise will often only cause distress and further confusion; it can be kinder to leave them lost in memory, if they are happier there than in reality.

I was told once that dementia can exaggerate pre-existing personality traits. Certainly, I have seen it make anxious people more anxious, but it can also make previously gentle people turn violent, or a rational mind turn paranoid. Gregory, normally as gentle a soul as you could ever meet, once trapped me against a closed bathroom door, shouting, with arm upraised, and Doris became convinced that every time we served a meal we were trying to poison her. Several of the men became preoccupied with sex. Jack, every time I had to go into his room, used to offer me £5 for my tights. I should have agreed; it would have been the quickest and easiest £5 I ever made. Mervyn would develop crushes on various female residents and members of staff and then stand, quite still and silent but far too close, behind their left shoulder. One night he followed Ava for her entire medication round; one after another we tried to usher him away, but he refused to budge. He was a tall, powerfully built man, and his looming presence was unnerving, the more so as he never said a word. But capping all were the tales the older staff used to tell of Cecil, who took delight in masturbating in front of them. Mercifully, by the time I arrived, he had been moved on. I learnt to cope with many new experiences at Ember Vale, but that might have been one experience too far.

The vast majority of the residents at Ember Vale were classed as 'living with dementia'. Of those, most 'lacked capacity', meaning that they were judged incapable of making their own complex decisions about care, finances, medical treatment and so on, and of *those*, a handful lived under Deprivation of Liberty Safeguards. This complicated and unpleasant piece of legislation, always referred to as DoLS, allows patients in care homes and hospitals to be restrained, supervised or medicated against their will, if this is judged 'in their best interest'. It can also be used to remove someone from their own home into a care home if this too is deemed best interest. The care home or hospital concerned must apply through the local authority for permission to deprive someone of their liberty in this way. Enforced isolation and confinement to one small bedroom for weeks at a time, however, is not subject to any external safeguarding at all.

Ember Vale, like most care homes, retained a small core of residents consisting of those who had been there for years and would be until they died. But there was also a fairly high turnover. A couple, like Marion, simply hated being there and fought tooth and nail to get out, or deliberately made so much trouble that they got themselves moved on. But these cases were rare. I can recall only one instance of someone leaving the care home to return to their own home. Everyone else left either on an undertaker's gurney or for another kind of institution. Ember Vale was not equipped, in either resources or staffing, to care for particularly difficult, disturbed or violent residents. Sometimes (as was the case with Cecil) these were 'sectioned' – committed to medical care under Section 2 of the Mental Health Act. When residents left, we were never told where they went or why, and I suppose we were not supposed to know. But everyone did.

I can still see the faces of those I cared for, and – mostly – remember their names. We were told, however, that we had to refer to residents not by name but by their room number. This was to protect their privacy – a laudable intention, but it made us uncomfortable; reducing people to numbers is hideously reminiscent of *Les Miserables*' Prisoner 24601, or the concentration camps of Nazi Germany. When residents' rooms were swapped around, which did not happen very often but often enough to make life awkward, the numbers system, inevitably, became confusing. So too with the two rooms reserved as isolation rooms (or 'rainbow rooms', as we were instructed to call them, because it sounds nicer and is suitably, fuzzily vague) for new incoming residents. Just as you had learnt which resident went with the room, they would be moved out into their own permanent room with another number and a new, different inmate would take their place.

When we *did* call residents by their own names, it was always by their Christian name. No Mr Smiths or Mrs Joneses, which is how I was brought up to refer to anyone in a generation above my own. The residents should, of course, have been asked how they would like to be addressed, but somehow nobody ever seemed to think of this. Some people prefer first names; when I was working as a volunteer at an Auckland retirement village, I had to school myself very hard to call Mr Prestwick Michael. (I never really succeeded. I could just about do it if I had to, but to me he was and always will be Mr Prestwick.) But others dislike the informality; my grandmother has always been Mrs Bloomfield to her multitude of cleaners (who never last very long before she sacks them as an unnecessary expense). And it always grated to hear my grandfather's carers cheerfully bellow out his first name, when his housekeeper, who had been with the family for thirty years and knew us almost as well as we knew ourselves, never called him anything other than Mr Olander. As for the people at Ember Vale, well, I am ashamed now to realise that I never knew which they preferred, because I never thought to ask them.

The image of the little old lady still holds powerful sway in the popular mindset. But at Ember Vale lived ladies – and gentlemen – both little and large, of all shapes, sizes and temperaments. Inadvertently, I once nearly tipped Cheryl out of her wheelchair; although visibly small and frail, she was so much lighter than I expected (wheelchairs, with or without an occupant, are usually heavy, unwieldy monsters) that I pushed off with completely the wrong amount of force. I learnt later that she weighed less than forty kilograms. At the other end of the scale (no pun intended) was Beryl, diabetic and classed as 'morbidly obese'. Incapable of walking, in her wheelchair she was more than twice my weight. She had a specially large bed and a specially large wheelchair and oh, how hard it was to manoeuvre them in her hatefully tiny little room. All the paint had been chipped off the bottom of her door and its frame because the wheelchair would only just fit through, and only then if it was perfectly straight. Swinging the weight round through ninety degrees off the corridor was so difficult that we usually hit the doorframe before having to reverse, straighten up and try again.

Most people at Ember Vale were in their eighties. A few had reached their nineties, and for a month we had Martin, who was one hundred, still in possession of his faculties, always particular in his habits and unfailingly courteous. He also had a terrifyingly iron will. He did not want to live any more, he certainly did not want to live at Ember Vale, and he simply stopped eating and drinking until he died. I sat beside him as he vomited, his body failing and shutting down, and he was courteous still. His swift, brutal decline shocked everyone, even those who had worked in care for years. He is one of those who haunts me still and probably always will.

Florence, who was physically tiny, in character larger than life and for over a year my bête noire before somehow becoming one of my favourites, did not quite make it to a hundred. I mourned this, because she was one of the very few who, even with clouded mind and physical infirmity, still managed to retain a certain zest for life. Outliers at the other end of the age range were Jack (he who offered me £5 for my tights), only in his fifties but admitted with early onset Alzheimer's, and Cindy, who was in her early seventies and therefore still young in elderly terms. Her own mother had only recently died, at the quite astonishing age of a hundred and four, so Cindy herself had potentially another thirty years' residence at Ember Vale.

Contemplating this prospect, and the sheer terrible monotony of thirty years in a care home, provoked a kind of awe-filled horror in those of us who had to look after her, for Cindy was the most miserable bugger I have ever met. She was much less incapacitated than she pretended, but it was a point of principle with her never to attempt the slightest thing for herself. She took active delight in being miserable and in making others miserable too. Possessed of a nasty vicious streak, she knew exactly how to needle or provoke staff already working under almost unbearable pressure. So in the mornings, which were always a hectic but doomed attempt to meet impossible time constraints, she would refuse to stand to enable the rotunda to be used to transfer her from bed to wheelchair. Whichever poor unfortunate had the job of getting her up that day would entreat, cajole, plead, all to no avail. This failing as it almost always did, a second carer would be hailed to take their turn. Depending on what mood Cindy decided to be in that morning, she would either get up like a lamb or remain lying there like an inert blob. In the evenings after tea, she would, without fail, suddenly develop an incurable 'stomach ache', which always led to a storm of shouting and crying. And whatever the time of day or night, she was always complaining, in a kind of whining mutter that was very hard to understand. She swore; she never looked anyone in the eye; she bitched about all the staff both behind our backs and to our faces. She was blatantly and outrageously racist. She never bothered to learn our names, or use them if she did know them, and would instead emit a whining cry of, "Carer! Carerrrrr!" whenever anyone had to pass by her room. She got under the skin of us all without exception, but she picked particularly on Lucille, who was of Jamaican heritage and whom I more than once found reduced to tears by Cindy's racist vitriol.

Dementia or no, Cindy was as sharp as a tack. I am quite sure that she *did* know all our names and merely pretended not to, just as she could stand perfectly well when she chose. There also appeared to be nothing whatsoever wrong with her short-term memory, for she would listen to the staff talking among themselves (we were not supposed to do this, but talking to each other was usually far preferable to attempting conversation with Cindy) and then refer back, days or even weeks later, to conversations we had not realised were being overheard. So, always catching me by surprise, she would ask me about the car (which had had two big bills on it within two months), the purchase of our house (everything that could go wrong did) and my baby (although when I brought him in she refused to hold him). If she ever saw me in mufti, she would also comment, favourably, on whatever I was wearing, and I would have to pick myself up off the floor after the shock of hearing something pleasant coming out of Cindy's loose-dentured mouth. These very rare occasions were the only time she gave us a glimpse of the woman that must have been hidden somewhere beneath the armour of bitterness and self-indulgent misery. I tried to seize on them and draw her out into conversation, but the spark of interest always faded like a spent match, and she would return to her moping and her muttering.

Nevertheless, Cindy regularly reminded me of what I did already know but, in the hurry and stress of a shift, all too easily forgot: it is wrong to assume those we care for do not understand. Such an attitude is common among those who interact with those suffering from dementia, not necessarily deliberately but because we do not take the time the person needs. It is wrong because it is rude but also because it is often simply *wrong*. Dementia does not make one stupid or insensible. Insight may not always be present, but its absence should not be assumed.

Sometimes those with dementia do possess an unexpected level of insight into their own condition. Struggling with fairly advanced dementia, my grandmother, one Christmas morning, dissolved into tears because she had forgotten to buy presents for all the family. "I used to be so on top of things," she sobbed, "so organised, and now my brain is letting me down... I've never known anything so horrible, *not even during the war...*" This incident seared itself into my memory and often I would return to it, mulling it over to wonder how the instability of dementia could outweigh the horrors of war. Confused and fragmentary snippets of family wartime history have come down to me from various family members. My grandmother, a small girl at the time, lived through the war in rural Austria, occupied by the Germans and subject to all the resulting restrictions, deprivations and fear. Food was often scarce and the winters harsh. Family and friends took diverging political paths. One uncle ended up in a concentration camp, where he fashioned jewellery out of bits of the barbed wire fence; the jewellery survived but he did not. Towards the end of the fighting, the German invasion was replaced by American occupation; one soldier pointed his gun at Grandma's father, the village baker, shouting that he was a member of the Nazi party. There was more, there must have been, but neither my grandmother nor her brother ever liked to speak much of those years. Yet the old terrors paled beside the newer ones of feeling at sea, adrift in a strange, ever-shifting world where she no longer had a reliable compass to guide her through the choppy waters.

Here is a scene you may have experienced or witnessed at some time or another, perhaps in the days when it was still permissible to talk face to face with the elderly instead of barricading them behind locked doors, Perspex screens or layers of hot plastic PPE. A daughter is with her elderly mother and happens to mention that it is a nice day, or that the cat has had a healthy litter of kittens, or that James came top of his class at school.

Mother: "Pardon?"

Daughter, slightly louder: "Lovely weather we're having!" (Or, "The cat had four kittens yesterday!" or, "James came top of his class in the end-of-year exams!")

Mother: "What? Can't hear you. Speak clearly!"

Daughter, much louder and slower: "LOVELY WEATHER!" (Or, "THE CAT HAD ITS KITTENS!" or, "JAMES CAME TOP OF HIS CLASS!")

Mother, recoiling: "All right! Don't shout! I'm not deaf, you know!"

Daughter, indignant: "I'm not shouting!"

Mother, righteous: "Yes you are!"

Daughter: "HUMPH!"

And each party sits in aggrieved and offended silence.

People quite understandably object to being shouted at in this way, for subtleties of speech are lost when the voice is raised. In the increased effort of communication, what is actually said is necessarily shorter and simpler. This has the unfortunate effect of making the shouter appear to talk down to the recipient. Instead of, "I'm not deaf, you know!" another common response is, "I'm not stupid, you know!" But what is the answer? Well, to check that any hearing aid batteries are working, I suppose. Beyond that, I don't know.

Many – not all – care home residents are hard of hearing. All the care staff unconsciously spoke in raised voices whenever on shift, and even then, we would have to repeat ourselves again and again and again. The masks were partly to blame for this: many people, even the young, rely on lip reading to fill in gaps misheard in speech. Wearing them, communication was infinitely harder than it would otherwise have been, especially in the communal areas where the background noise usually consisted of the television, the radio, the call bells, the telephone ringing, the telephone being answered, Cindy shouting, Florence banging and Sinead diddly-diddly-deeing. I particularly struggled to make myself understood. I knew how to project my voice – I taught for years, and a strong throat is essential for this, especially when trying to control a class of five-year-old budding ballerinas. But people tell me I am softly spoken, and my accent, tone and cadences of speech were very different from those I was working with. I suppose it was simply harder for residents to tune in to me than to the rest of the staff, because my speech was different.

I had many a battle royale with Damian to make myself understood. Damian really was deaf, at least as long as his hearing aids were out. With them in, he was selectively deaf. He could hear other people, if they spoke loudly. But he could not hear me at all, no matter how I bellowed. After one episode of shouting myself red in the face, I came upon Lynn doubled over with laughter. Apparently, whenever I was in Damian's room, I could be heard all over the building and, she said, "Normally you're so quiet and polite!" I was mortified, but what was I to do? Damian, I think, simply did not like me, a feeling which I have to confess was mutual. Making me shout seemed for him a perverse kind of game (I suppose there was little enough other entertainment on offer, so fair enough). But it was not a game that I enjoyed, and I grew to dread going into his room.

Damian was deaf. Sinead sang, "Diddly diddly dee, diddly diddly dee," on repeat, and every night on going to bed would ask, "Do you love me?" Edith, who had been in the wartime Auxiliary Territorial Service, was unfailingly upright and as smartly turned out as she had been seventy-five years before. Margery was always cheerful and always singing, in a slow, cracked, agonisingly tuneless voice that nevertheless brought pleasure to those who heard it. Cindy was relentlessly miserable. Christopher worked tapestry. Jack asked all of us in turn for our tights. Gregory tried to reorganise the plumbing. Ethel was everyone's favourite, because she was so lovely and easy-going. Shyla was a Catholic, and for this regarded by some members of the staff as if she came from outer space. Ellen, who truly made you feel that life was a vale of tears, was always begging the Lord to take her; so far, He had declined, presumably because heaven's undiluted bliss would be undiluted no longer once she arrived. Angela tried to get out every night: "I've got to go and look after the horses, you idiot!" Stella always had a book in her hand and read almost as fast as I did. Victoria walked the corridors half the night and then slept half the day, rising only to resume walking, dragging her quilt behind her along the corridor. Cheryl acted like the lady of the manor, always imperious, never satisfied, and drove us all to distraction.

Many people assume that the elderly are all the same, a grey and amorphous array. Dementia, depression and the imposition of a rigid, institutionalised routine can appear to dampen or deaden personality, but the reality is of course that the elderly are as diverse as the rest of us. All the residents of Ember Vale had their own quirks, tics and traits. Occasionally these demonstrations of personality asserted themselves against the daily routine, usually leading to a lot more work for us but welcomed nonetheless as poignant reminders of humanity and individualism. A disproportionate number of these events seemed to involve the toilets and fluids of one kind or another.

One unforgettable evening Gregory decided to replumb one of the downstairs bathrooms. In working life, he had been a carpenter, and quite often he would wander the home knocking and banging on the walls and skirtings. Everyone was used to this and let him get on with it, except when he tried to take doors off their hinges; the fact that he still had all his fingers intact was a minor miracle. So, when he was noticed moseying around the bathroom, nobody took much notice – which was in hindsight a mistake, but there were never enough staff to keep on top of things. We were always running around putting out metaphorical fires instead of catching them in time to prevent sparks taking hold.

In this case, however, it was not fire that transpired but water. Somehow, Gregory managed to wrench off the pipe beneath the sink as well as blocking the toilet with handful upon handful of paper towels. The result was a flood of Biblical proportions and an unholy stench. By the time the stopcock had been located and turned off, the water, mingling with the brown overflow from the toilet, was several inches deep on the floor. Gregory, soaked through but quite happy, was most put out at being led away from the scene. The flood took hours to clean up, by which time all the staff involved were also wet through, and the bathroom was out of use for days while the results of Gregory's handiwork were repaired and painted over.

True friendships among the residents were rare – partly because few had anything in common beyond age, infirmity and shared lodgings, partly because many were no longer capable of forming new relationships, and partly because a two-year cycle of individual isolation and segregation was not conducive to forming social bonds. But, human nature being what it is, unassailable even by dementia, groups and attachments did form. At mealtimes we were supposed to ask where each person wanted to sit, but without fail, everyone always sat in exactly the same place – and woe betide anyone who took another person's place. A couple of the ladies flirted, mildly, with the men (women outnumbered men in the home by at least three to one). Tiny little Georgina attached herself to Ethel, who good-naturedly took on the role of protector and performed it with heroic patience, even when Georgina took to following her everywhere like a little shadow. But in general, the bonds between resident and carer were stronger than those between resident and resident.

Of course we were not supposed to have favourites, and equally, of course, everyone did. Top of everyone's list was Ethel, who was the only long-standing resident not suffering from some form of dementia. She walked, slowly and painfully, with a frame, and she needed some help with washing and dressing, but otherwise she remained stubbornly independent, and her mind was perfectly clear. I often wondered how she could be so content in such a place, for she was a clever woman and had lived a busy and varied life. She never married and had no children or surviving family, but she did not seem lonely. But Ethel, unlike me, was expert in Making the Best of Things and Just Getting on with Life. Also unlike me, she saw the best in people by default, which was of course why everyone liked her so much. But she was not some paragon of angelic virtue. She never said anything – or at least, not much, and only very discreetly – but I knew perfectly well that she found some of the more difficult residents as trying as we did. She knew all our names and never failed to thank us – two small-seeming gestures that meant the world. She was interested in all of us and in our lives outside the care home.

She was also, apparently, something of a petrol head. To get to work, I drove David's car, a red and black Mini Cooper Sport; it had a throaty growl, a powerful engine, and it looked very out of place in the care home car park. From her seat in the lounge, Ethel saw me drive up one day and quizzed me with keen interest about the car, how it ran and what it was like to drive. She herself had owned several good cars, delighting in their power and the freedom of the open road. Often after that she would greet me with, "And how's your lovely car?" She commiserated with me about the price of petrol and the unlucky, unforeseen bills. From the car itself, we progressed to driving and travelling, and I told her how we would drive at weekends to go walking in the hills, where in the space and open air we could forget for a little while about Covid, lockdowns and the care home. She sympathised with this too, and every Friday she asked if I was going walking that weekend and would reminisce about hill holidays she herself had enjoyed many years before.

Ethel, like many of the residents, enjoyed the television, which became for many almost their sole link with the outside world. She particularly liked the quiz shows, although her tastes were eclectic: she also liked murder mysteries (this was another topic of conversation, as I can eat my way through murder mysteries with an ease surpassed only by the efficiency with which David consumes a box of chocolates), *Antiques Roadshow* and *The Repair Shop*, and *Countryfile*. And every Sunday without fail she would watch *Songs of Praise*. Although she was not outwardly religious, she always knew all the hymns and would hum along to them, beating out the time on the armrest of her chair.

Apart from *Songs of Praise*, religiosity was not much in evidence, certainly not on a communal level. In pre-Covid days, Sunday services had been held every month or so, but these were halted during the lockdowns and never reintroduced. The care plans included space for religious affiliation to be recorded, most people's saying either *Church of England* or *None Specified*; the split was roughly equal. A couple of residents were notably devout: Ellen, who had a crucifix above her bed, and Stella, whose substantial collection of books included several of a religious nature and a slim black Bible, which she was holding as she died.

Shyla was the only non-white resident and the only one who was a Catholic. Cindy commented on the former and Maddie, one of the seniors, on the latter; by their tone both managed to imply that Shyla must therefore also have two heads. At first, I was rather pleased by the prospect of a fellow Catholic joining the home. I thought it might be a good way into conversation; I believe I also had visions of her wanting us to pray the Rosary together, although given the time constraints we all worked under, this was an absurd delusion from the start. Anyway, in the event, Shyla turned out to be a Catholic, yes, but also to believe in black magic; she also took a near-instant dislike to me and refused to let me anywhere near her. And so that was that.

(I worried at first at this dislike, wondering what I had done or said to earn it, but it soon spread to other members of staff as well, so that on some shifts we were all on Shyla's blacklist and she would either have to decide which of us she disliked the least, or put herself to bed, which she categorically refused to do, or wait for the night staff.)

On the inside of my right wrist is a silvery-brown scar, fading now, but for a long time it stood out against the skin. This is a memento of Florence, permanent testimony to her dislike of taking a shower. Her aversion to washing was rather extreme, although many of the residents did not like being showered; Florence merely took this dislike to the next level. She was one of the home's biggest characters, despite being less than four feet tall; she was noisy, messy, violent and occasionally affectionate; I first hated and then loved her, and of all the deaths, hers was probably the one I most mourned.

Florence had no teeth, next to no hair except a kind of white fluffy tonsure, and spent all day every day ensconced in one of the comfy armchairs, under a blanket which she usually pulled up to her chin so that only her head peeked out. Hunched in her chair, muttering and cackling to herself, she resembled nothing so much as one of Macbeth's witches. The blanket was usually liberally adorned with porridge, mashed vegetables or smeared chocolate, for despite having no teeth, she was still a hearty eater. If she was particularly frustrated that morning, she would throw her tea down the blanket for good measure and then smile serenely at the sighs and exclamations of the staff. She did a lot of shouting, some singing and a fair bit of pretending to be a brass band, banging on her table and calling out, "Barum-pum-pum, barum-pum-pum, bam!" And when she had to be showered, she screamed blue murder.

Each care staff member was assigned two or three residents for whom they had to assume particular responsibility, including ensuring that they had a full bath or shower at least once a week. Shortly after I arrived, Maddie, with a smug smirk, assigned me 'two nice easy assistance of ones'. Assistance of one, also known as a 'single', meant that the resident could mobilise with the support of only one carer as opposed to two. The smirk meant that the residents were not easy ones, and that I knew they were not easy ones, and that Maddie knew that I knew they were not easy ones. One of my two was Georgina, who in herself was as meek as a lamb but came with a daughter who (lockdowns notwithstanding) was always popping up to cause trouble. ("You, what's-your-name, carer. Has Mum eaten today? Has Mum drunk today? Why doesn't Mum's top match her skirt? Are you sure that's Mum's bra? Mum's hair doesn't look right. When did Mum last have a shower? When did Mum last have her hair washed? Are Mum's hearing aids in? Mum's bed hasn't been made properly. Mum looks hot. Mum looks cold. Mum looks flustered. Are you *sure* Mum's eaten today? Are you *sure* Mum's drunk today? Is Mum's food organic like I requested? Mum! Mum! Have you eaten today? Have you drunk today? Mum! Mum! Can you hear me? Carer, are you *sure* Mum's hearing aids are in? Well, why aren't they working? It's disgraceful, disgraceful. I need to speak to the senior. No, I can't wait. I'll speak to the manager instead. Outrageous, all the money we're paying. Carer! Carer! I haven't finished.") The other was Florence.

I had to shower Florence each week, and so – dutifully, grimly – I did shower Florence each week. It was an exercise which I dreaded for days beforehand and left me limp afterwards. I always did it as early in the week as possible, usually on a Monday, so that it was got out of the way. If there were new staff on shift, I had to warn them beforehand that, contrary to what they might suspect from what they were about to hear, I was not actually murdering Florence in the bathroom. She writhed and wriggled, twisted and turned; she slapped and hit and scratched and bit; and she screamed and screamed and screamed. The bathroom always ended up swimming with water and covered in talcum powder; between the physical exertion and the hot steaminess of the bathroom, my tunic would be soaked in sweat and shower water. Strangely, once she had her nighty on and was helped into bed, Florence always quietened down, becoming mild-mannered and demure; sometimes she even murmured a thank you and tried to kiss me goodnight. But, wet and exhausted, I remained stonily unmoved by these demonstrations of affection.

One night Florence scratched me so hard on the wrist that it drew blood from deep lacerations. I tried to hide this, knowing that if it was spotted, I would be made to fill in a long-winded and completely useless behaviour chart in addition to the rest of the usual paperwork. But the blood on my tunic was something of a giveaway: "You'll have to fill in a behaviour chart for her." Groan. Fortunately, Marge, the senior on duty, had the tact (unusual for her) not to suggest that it was my own fault for failing to keep Florence's nails short. I did occasionally try to clean, cut and file them, but it would have been easier to trim the nails of a tiger.

For months, Florence and I waged a war of wills. Then one Monday in early January, I went to shower her, even more depressed than usual. I had spent most of the Christmas holidays working on a job application for a research fellow's position at the London Globe. It was exactly the kind of job I wanted; I was qualified for it; I had spent hours working on the application and those to whom I had shown it and requested feedback from said it was strong. And it did not even pass the shortlisting stage.

I got Florence through the shower in morose silence on my part and the usual sound effects on hers. Afterwards I knelt on the floor in front of her in order to rub cream onto her legs, whereupon she screeched that I was a bugger and started slapping my face. I put up an arm to ward off the blows and something suddenly snapped. All my years of hard work, plans and ambitions, hopes and dreams, all had come to this – trapped in a horrendous job in a foul-smelling prison, with a hateful old witch verbally and physically assaulting me. Still kneeling on the floor, I burst into a passion of angry, bitter crying. It was one of the lowest moments of my life. I was crying not merely about the job but for the loss of everything else: family, home and career, my self-esteem and self-respect, the baby I had miscarried a month before, the complete, utter injustice of things.

A miracle happened. Florence began to comfort me. Her hands began gently to caress my hair and her angry shouting changed to soft soothing. *There, there, don't cry, everything's all right.* So many times at Ember Vale I had tried to comfort people in this way, and now, in a complete reversal of roles, a ninety-eight-year-old dementia sufferer was doing it to me. We were both trapped, she within the frailties of age, I in a job I loathed, each isolated in misery. But in that moment, barriers fell away, and a connection was formed. Everything was not all right, but we reached out to each other and helped one another.

After a while, I stopped crying. I helped Florence into bed, tucked her up, kissed her on the cheek and turned off the light on my way out to continue the rest of my rounds. If anyone noticed my tear-stained face and red, swollen nose, they said nothing. The mask hid it, I suppose.

I will always be grateful to Florence for helping me in that moment, and I became very fond of her. I no longer minded the screaming and the lashing out. I knew exactly how she felt and, albeit in a less violent way, I knew that at home I was taking out the same feelings of frustration on poor long-suffering David. In her less disturbing moments, Florence still liked a glass of sherry and still possessed a surprisingly good sense of humour; she liked to laugh, and I found myself wondering what she had been like in youth. In the right mood she could, I discovered, be very affectionate, seizing my hand and covering it with kisses. When one of the other staff told her I was pregnant – this time with a baby that stayed put – she stroked my thickening waist and jabbered away in a stream of excited babble of which the only intelligible word was 'baby'.

I promised her I would bring the baby in after it was born, but Florence never met him. When I did bring him in a few months later, there was an interloper in Florence's chair, for she had died shortly after I went on maternity leave. I hope it was quick; she must have gone downhill fast, for the day I left she was singing out in fine form, installed as ever in what was always known as Florence's chair. I saw her death on the WhatsApp handover group, a simple, bald statement of fact – *Passed away peacefully 3:35am. Rest in peace* – and felt indescribably sad.

4

STAFF

Care home staff in this country work for minimum wage, in appalling conditions, under the most ridiculous pressures and expectations, on shift patterns that are often illegal, continually overshadowed in the media and the public perception by their much richer and much-lauded cousin, the NHS.

Small wonder, then, that the sector is both chronically understaffed and has an extremely high turnover rate.

If Ember Vale was ever properly staffed while I worked there, I must have blinked and missed it. There was a continuous parade of new staff and new faces who would appear and then disappear again, often before we had time to learn their names. Quite a few left after just one shift, appalled at what the job entailed. A few more left after a week or two, once the reality of the long, antisocial hours for pathetic pay had sunk in. One or two simply never started at all and I was to learn that this was not uncommon. It was to do with the jobseeker's benefit, where people had to show they were looking for work in order to keep receiving payments but apparently were not obliged to take up work if offered it. After working at the home for about six weeks, I was astonished to discover that, by virtue of this length of service, I was classed as one of the 'old' employees. This meant I had to train newcomers, which I disliked doing, having received next to no training myself.

Shifts were filled by people working overtime, or by people working outside their contract – domestic staff on care, for example. Occasionally, when all else failed, we had agency staff, which actually made more work, because they were unfamiliar with the home's routines and residents and could not be left unsupervised. Quite often, shifts were not filled at all. A fully staffed shift, an entity almost as mythical as Pegasus, was supposed to consist of seven people: the senior (properly called the care team leader) and six care staff, who were assigned one to each of the four corridors and two as 'floats', one upstairs and one down. In reality, this almost never happened. Mostly we had just one float; quite often we worked with just four care staff, and there were times when we did it with three. Extra shifts or hours over our contracts would sometimes appear as if by magic on our rotas, but more usually Lynn would run around the home clutching the red file that held the printed roster, trying to beg, bribe or bully people into covering hours. I learnt very quickly not to answer my phone on days off, but a pleading message would always be left on my voicemail. I knew it by heart without having to play it back: "Hello, Eleanor, it's Marge calling from Ember Vale. When you get this, can you give me a call back?" I never did. I hated being hounded in this way, but it forced me to toughen up. For the first time in my life, I learnt to say no and, as time went by, to do so without a twinge of people-pleasing guilt.

We always seemed particularly, suspiciously, short on weekends and bank holidays. If Lynn had not managed to cover these shifts before she left on Friday afternoons, the job would fall to the seniors. It was a task they hated. I understood why but resented the pressure and arm twisting that some applied. One day, Marge, desperate, actually barricaded me into the office with the meds trolley, brandishing the rota and attempting a bit of psychological manipulation. "Hello, Eleanor." (Unconvincing smile.) "Can you cover some shifts this weekend?"

"No."

"We're really short!"

"Nothing new there. No."

"You could use the extra money!"

"True. But no."

"I'm working overtime!"

"Your choice. No."

"The home can't be understaffed!"

(Snort.) "No."

"I don't want to have to call the agency!"

"I don't care. No."

"Please!"

"No."

Ironically, if she had not physically blocked me from leaving the office, I would probably have caved in and agreed. But the attempt at intimidation was so ridiculous that I was roused at last into defiance. I won. I had learnt the power of no. It was liberating and exhilarating, and I wished I had learnt it years ago.

Leila worked a lot of overtime, but she would never agree to it without first demanding to know who was already working the shift; then, depending on whether she liked them or not, she would either agree or decline. The senior always demurred at this – "The roster is confidential!" But of course they always capitulated. The shift had to be filled, and as long as it was filled, nobody cared how.

The idea of the roster being confidential was silly anyway and utterly pointless – how can who you are working with on any given shift be kept confidential? The red folder was supposed to live locked up in Lynn's office, but it spent far more time in one of the office cupboards we all had access to, or out on the desk, where it was frequently left by a harassed senior. Here we would shamelessly pore over it to see who was working with whom and to bargain for swaps. I never agreed to a swap unless I could rely completely on my opposite number, for if they failed to turn up to cover your shift, you were technically responsible for taking it on again yourself.

I was contracted for twenty-eight hours a week, which equated to four shifts. Everyone, whether or not they did official overtime, ended up working over their contracted hours – without pay, of course. To begin with, the shifts were not seven hours long but seven hours and twenty minutes; this was to allow for a twenty-minute unpaid break. Breaks, especially on the busy morning shift, were something of a joke; nobody ever managed to take them at their allocated time and sometimes the shift was so busy they never happened at all, or were cut short. Despite the warnings of more experienced staff, this happened to me several times, but after a few weeks I learnt, as with the overtime, to put my foot down. If we had been paid properly to begin with, if we had been treated by the company as human beings instead of expendable commodities, if the shifts had been properly staffed so that we were not continually trying to meet impossible targets, I would not have minded. But however hard we worked, it was never enough, so I saw no point in running myself even further into the ground for ever smaller returns. I always took my twenty minutes, and I always told new staff to make sure they took theirs.

Then there was the paperwork, always referred to simply as 'the books'. This in total was supposed to take twenty minutes per shift – what a joke! On a full corridor of ten residents, that meant two minutes' writing time per resident. Two minutes in which to complete the two-hourly observations (always called 'ticks'), write a summary of the individual's personal care, behaviour, activities and well-being for the day, record any creams or ointments administered, complete the shower chart if one was given, fill in the hated food and fluid chart and complete, if required, any behaviour charts or incident forms. Twenty minutes my foot. The paperwork for one single resident could easily take that long on its own. Lynn was always promising iPads and a shift to digital paperwork to speed things up, but they never materialised. (Probably too expensive.) Several people took the paperwork into the staff room to complete on their break, which we were forbidden to do, but then we were also forbidden to leave unless the paperwork was done. I refused to do paperwork on my break, and I refused to stay behind after a shift to finish it. I wrote fast and was naturally concise, so I usually managed to get it done on time, but conscientious Lucille would often stay behind after a shift for forty-five minutes or more to finish her books. I admired her for it and helped her where I could but – my good-girl reputation notwithstanding – could not imitate her zeal.

Thrown together in this fashion, leaving a sleeping household in the mornings and returning in the evenings well after the end of the conventional working day, working weekends when normal people were enjoying a whole two days off, it often felt as if we saw more of each other than of our own families, and more of the care home than of our own homes. Working in such close proximity, always under ceaseless pressure, tensions and tempers inevitably flared, personalities clashed and people rubbed each other up the wrong way. The staff were overwhelmingly female, and a good deal of bitching went on. I have no idea what was said about me behind my back, but often I found myself playing the familiar role of piggy in the middle: two different people would come up to me at different times to complain, discreetly or loudly according to their nature, about the other. I would listen gravely and sympathise with each and wonder what it was about me that apparently, whatever life situation I found myself in, made me people's chosen confidant.

I got on pretty well with almost everyone, not because of enhanced social skills (ha!) but because I kept my head down and was a hard worker. The cardinal crime at Ember Vale was to be a shirker, and those branded with this label were never welcomed or accepted. I got a lot of ribbing for my accent, my background ("You're so posh!") and my frocks and heeled shoes, but I think I was respected for my work. In return, I greatly respected most of my colleagues, many of whom worked longer hours than I did, had families to raise and mortgages to pay on minimum wage, and yet still managed to turn up day after day with a smile and a sense of humour, even if the latter was often of the gallows variety.

Being no saint, an admission of reality that will come as no surprise to my husband and family, certain people did rub me up the wrong way. Usually, though, they were universally disliked by the other staff as well, which somehow made me feel less of a terrible person – I suppose because it allowed me to feel it wasn't me, it was them. False logic this may be, but working at Ember Vale, you took comfort where it was offered.

Gemma, one of the seniors, was the only person I didn't get on with when everyone else did; she was widely revered for her length of service. We got off to a bad start, as when she first encountered me at the door she looked me up and down as if I were something the cat had dragged in. I was markedly taller than her, but she managed to make me feel about two feet high and two years old. With the residents, she was sweetness itself and seemed genuinely caring, but whenever I was in view, she either coldly ignored me or criticised me to the skies. I have no idea why she disliked me and didn't care, for I returned her disdain as heartily as she gave it. When I heard she was leaving to take up another position I was relieved, but Fate wasn't letting her go before playing one final trick on us both. A leaving party was organised for her to which we were all summoned; I dutifully attended, but only because I was rostered on for that shift anyway and therefore couldn't get out of it. Lynn made a speech, at which she wept, Gemma wept and many of the staff wept while I remained stonily dry-eyed. Lynn then hugged Gemma (farewell, Covid protocol!); Gemma fervently hugged her back; and this continued all around the room, Gemma hugging staff and residents alike and wiping tears away between each one. When she got to me, she hesitated, dry-eyed. She clearly did not want to hug me, I certainly did not want to hug her, and we both knew exactly what the other was thinking. But clearly, too, she felt it would look bad if she did not, so eventually she leaned in stiffly; I returned the hug with as little contact as possible; and she moved quickly on. At least she did not have to wipe her eyes dry before approaching the next candidate.

Leadership by some of the seniors was poor. The hallmarks of a good leader are a.) to lead by example, and b.) not to demand your staff do something you yourself won't, basic rules of management which were frequently breached. Certain seniors were lazy, doing as little work as possible and then blaming the care staff when the shift did not run smoothly. In doing so, they lost respect and, with it, their authority, setting in motion a vicious cycle: everyone became resentful and harassed and the shift went from bad to worse. By contrast, the better shifts were bearable because of who was running them. We were constantly being exhorted by Lynn to communicate better with each other, but improved day-to-day leadership would have gone a long way to improving morale. In fairness to the seniors, an extra 50p an hour was, as Ava once bitterly pointed out, poor compensation for the extra responsibility (and the extra paperwork, which some busied themselves with ad infinitum). Several of the long-standing staff refused to undergo the training to become care team leaders for this very reason.

The buck always stopped with the care staff, and a very unpleasant stopping place it was too. It stopped at the end of a long chain, beginning with the Care Quality Commission (CQC), who hounded and threatened NG, who hounded and threatened the area managers, who hounded and threatened Lynn, who hounded and threatened the seniors, who hounded and threatened us. Full staff meetings did happen, but more often, Lynn liked to closet herself with each of the separate teams: seniors, kitchen and domestic. Lastly, she would instruct the care staff to attend what was simply an exercise in being blamed for all the home's woes. We were summoned (unpaid) to these meetings on a semi-regular basis. The seniors and other staff were never present, so, although I did once or twice stand up to point out that most of our perceived failings were a direct result of the impossible conditions we worked under, I spoke into a vacuum and was summarily dismissed by Lynn. The other care staff agreed with me, and said so, but nobody else wanted to hear it, and I never bothered speaking up again. It was pointless.

These meetings always followed the same format: Lynn would gravely inform us which of the CQC's impossibly tortuous standards we had failed this time and remind us that we were thereby putting the home at risk of failing an inspection and therefore (never stated but always implied) of her losing her job. Then she would pass on the 'feedback' garnered from the other meetings. The seniors said that we did not empty the dining room fast enough after meals. The kitchen staff said that we did not clear the tables properly after meals. The domestic staff said that we left bedrooms and lounges in a disgusting state. For form's sake, we were asked if there was anything we wanted to raise; few people ever bothered, because there was no point. (Leila, however, always asked for a pay increase, a request always greeted by sniggers of derision from the rest of us.) The meeting then concluded by a drill in hand washing or donning and doffing PPE; the number of times we were made to do this, while Lynn stood gravely by with clipboard and checklist, was quite absurd. Still, I can assure you that I know how to wash my hands. I can also assure you that nobody ever follows to the letter each prescribed step for doffing PPE, because if they did, they would a.) never do anything else and b.) have hands and arms red-raw from washing and sanitising.

Every so often, Lynn spotted some egregious breach of policy, or, more likely, had one sanctimoniously reported to her by one of the visiting professionals, usually the district nurses. This set off a whirlwind of banging doors and thudding foot-strikes as she marched up and down the home, sweeping up staff and depositing them in the office. Here, while the rest of the care staff were rounded up, we waited to hear what we had done this time; then the door was solemnly shut upon us and Lynn launched upon what became a familiar dressing-down – a Terrible Thing had come to her attention, she was very disappointed in us, if an inspector had seen the Terrible Thing, we would have failed immediately – we had to do better; we had to communicate better; never forget that we were a *team*, etc, etc.

Despite everything, I genuinely liked Lynn and respected her highly. The unrealistic pressures of the work were not of her making but imposed in obedience to higher powers. Caught between a rock and a hard place, sandwiched between CQC and her frequently mutinous, ever-changing staff, she had an impossibly difficult role. Not for the world would I have wanted her job. She was paid a great deal more than we were, but she worked hard for it, putting in long weekday hours; even when she was at home or on leave, she had to respond to the latest crisis. When we were desperately short-staffed, she rolled up her sleeves and pitched in alongside the care staff, not finding this beneath her as some of the seniors did. She was larger than life, loud and often impatient, but somehow, she always managed to be heartily cheerful, or at least to give the appearance of it; as an impossible Eeyore myself, I admired and envied this trait. Although the staff often grumbled about her, she did care about them. I trusted her, and it was her kindness and understanding that propped me up through my wobbliest moments.

Day to day the staff bickered, squabbled and complained about each other, but when it mattered they supported each other, in a sturdy, no-nonsense way that was a great deal more useful than society's fondness for platitudes of thoughts and prayers. Those who drove gave lifts to those who did not. A uniform was lent to me when my own took weeks to arrive. Anyone going on maternity leave was treated like royalty. A collection was always taken up for those who had been bereaved, and I experienced from many people a quiet generosity that often seemed in inverse proportion to their rate of pay. On what should have been my wedding day, I was rostered on for the morning shift, which passed without anything out of the ordinary until lunchtime, when we were all summoned to the dining room. Already glum, my heart sank further: what had we done now? I tried to hide at the back, next to the kitchen door. Out of this popped one of the kitchen staff, bearing a cake which was presented to a very astonished me while everyone looked on; meanwhile, Marge waxed lyrically about my cancelled wedding until, unable to hide my blushes anywhere else, I tried to hide them behind the cake. When, a few weeks later, I did go off to get married – the wedding pulled together in three weeks, slipping semi-miraculously into a brief period of lockdown easing; none of my family could be there, and I walked alone down the aisle – I was sent on my way with flowers, chocolates, money and a card signed by most of the staff. In spite of the cake episode, I was again utterly astonished.

At Christmas, everyone except the few grinches took part in a Secret Santa, and on Christmas Day, I opened a heavy package to find the complete works of Shakespeare, smartly bound in black and gold. I valued the book highly, and it now has pride of place on my living room bookshelf, but more than anything, I valued the thought and care which had gone into its choosing. I knew who had given it, and tried, very badly, to express how much it meant to me. But I could not find the words to explain how much it mattered, nor why. My own books, my most prized possessions and the escape portal from the tedium of daily life, languished twelve thousand miles away in my own little room at home while I worked unhappily in a job a million miles away from the world of academia and theatre I loved. Above and beyond its literary pleasures, that book offered hope of better things to come and stood as a reminder that I had not quite lost all I had worked for.

Before my first baby was born, Leila and Ava organised a baby shower for me. A long table in the Rose and Crown was taken over by people popping in before their shift, after their shift or on their day off. Lynn and Amelia, the assistant manager, came in on their lunch break. I was overwhelmed, quite literally, by a shower of presents: I had to recruit help carrying them to the car, where they completely filled the boot, the two back seats and the passenger seat. I drove off conscious of having failed utterly in thanks, surrounded by enough nappies to last a month, several little clothes and outfits (including three cardigans handknitted by Justine), a goodly supply of toys, spoons and beakers and a collection of £70 in cash. I piled everything up in the lounge when I got home and almost cried to look at it (let's blame the pregnancy hormones).

When that baby was nine weeks old, I took him into the home, wearing one of the outfits he had been given, bundled up against the December sleet in one of Justine's cardigans. For a good couple of hours, he was purred over and doted on and passed round from hand to hand. I smiled to see the pleasure he brought, but at the same time, my heart ached that work should meet my child before my parents did. I will never forgive the New Zealand government for closing the border so harshly and for so long, ensuring that my family missed my wedding and the arrival of their first grandchild, the two happiest, scariest, most important events of my life. Yet, in many ways, I was lucky. I had wonderful in-laws, and at work I had found friends.

"Drink," Leila said, thrusting towards me a mug filled with hot soup purloined from the kitchen. In vain I protested that I was not hungry; she merely stood there, holding out the mug, until I gave in and meekly accepted it. I *was* hungry, but – more to the point – it was useless arguing with her. Leila was Romanian; she was sturdy and strong; she worked fast and furiously; she rivalled me in impatience and in stubbornness; and hidden beneath a gruff exterior, she had a heart of gold. "I cannot remember your name," she announced airily when we first met. "I call you Sunshine." And Sunshine I was, at least until I somehow became Sweetheart instead. I was scared of her at first, and I think she thought I was some delicate little thing who would run, shuddering, from the job after a day or two. I shuddered, but I also stayed. And I worked hard. It was this that won her approval, and from there I soon discovered sympathy and kindness, always delivered in an understated, off-hand manner; after long years living in Britain, she typified the British dislike of fuss and emotion.

Her family in Romania, mine in New Zealand, neither of us knowing when we would meet again; we had this in common, rarely acknowledging it directly but drawing some secret support from shared experience. Strange ties the pandemic formed; one of the residents once innocently asked if I was Leila's daughter, a question which tickled my Romanian friend mightily. But in fact, she did look out for me, not quite in a motherly way but more in the manner of a solid and earthy guardian angel. Once she discovered I was pregnant, I actually had to hide from her in order to get done any work that she considered remotely heavy (pretty much everything except the paperwork). Otherwise, she would pop up, tutting and swearing, and take over whatever I was doing, leaving me to trail meekly and quite superfluously in her wake. She made sure I was fed and watered; she forced me to take breaks; she helped me with my books; and she gave me the best workplace laugh I ever had when she told me earnestly one winter morning about the reindeer that had visited her garden while she enjoyed a glass of after-work cider.

Drink was universal as a coping mechanism. During lockdowns, with the pubs closed, some staff congregated in the car park instead for a bring-your-own booze-up. Throughout the intermittent easing of restrictions, the Rose and Crown, the pub around the corner from the home, must have got good patronage from both Ember Vale and the home next door, Manfred House. I never went, being far too shy and always anxious to get away from work and its environs. I did drink, though. Somehow, a ritual developed where, coming home after the late shift, David would hand me a gin and tonic as I walked through the door; as time went on, they became progressively stiffer. Sometimes he had to make me a second before I could relax enough to sleep. This was, of course, dangerous, but I did not recognise it at the time; I wanted only to forget.

Most of the staff also smoked, and swearing was ubiquitous as a milder form of stress relief. Leila, at the end of every shift, would announce, "I bugger off home now." If the shift had been worse than usual, it was, "I fuckoffsky now." I did not smoke and did not swear either, though I often felt like it. This restraint, the result of habit and upbringing rather than virtue, was chalked up as another of my faintly endearing, faintly mockable eccentricities, along with my RP accent and the fact that I had a university degree.

Actually, I had three university degrees, but never mentioned them and disliked them being referred to. For some reason, most people assumed that, in pre-Covid times, I had worked as an actor (ironic, since I cannot manage to give even a simple presentation without descending into a visible mass of nerves). One resident's daughter thought I had worked in musical theatre (also ironic, since I cannot sing) and said, patronisingly, "Oh, you must be so anxious to get back to it!" I never bothered to correct these misapprehensions. The world in which I now worked was so far removed from the rarefied atmosphere of academia that my halcyon days of reading, writing and research seemed only a dim and distant dream, vanished beyond reach or recall. When wiping someone's arse, it doesn't matter if you have a PhD or left school at fourteen. Dealing with shit and piss and death made us all the same.

A paradoxical and two-fold shame also kept me silent – embarrassment that I had, in comparison to most of my colleagues, so many advantages in education and upbringing, and humiliation that those advantages had led me only to this hot and smelly hellhole. Despite being on good terms with most of my workmates, and genuinely close to a few of them, I often felt very lonely. The only girl (we were all girls, no matter how old or young) hailing from a similar background was Celine, bright, cheerful and outgoing. She was finishing her undergraduate degree during the first lockdown, with plans to go on to a master's and then PhD. With the universities closed and all classes cancelled or shifted online, she applied to work at the home in order, as she said, to stop herself going crazy with boredom and to save up for a new car. She was the only one who understood the straddling of two utterly different worlds and the difficulties of reconciling them. But she was a few years younger than I and at the beginning of her studies rather than the end of them, and when the universities reopened, she dropped her hours to bank work and then resigned completely. I watched her go with regret and envy; doors would open for her along her chosen path while all mine seemed not only slammed shut but locked and triple-bolted.

Celine, with her cheery nature, made any shift better. So did James, nicknamed by Gemma (he was one of her favourites) the 'grasshopper', because he seemed to do everything in an irrepressible, good-natured flurry. He was one of the very few male staff and, of those, one of the even fewer, perhaps the only one, who worked well alongside the women. Everyone liked him because he was unfailingly cheerful, always polite, and, without being pretentious or old-fashioned, a gentleman. He too was unusual among the staff for having a degree; like Celine, he had worked at the home as a student and returned to it after the first lockdown caused him to lose his graduate job in marketing. If he resented this, he rarely showed it.

Celine and James were the cheery ones. Leila was (often unfairly) the grumpy one. I was the quiet one, Lynn the loud one. Jess had a sense of humour so dry that only when you knew her well (and sometimes not even then) could you tell when she was joking. Justine, who gave me what little training I received, had worked in care for over thirty years; she was formidable, as tough as old boots, and I never quite stopped being scared of her. Alyssa called everyone babe, never did any work and was usually to be found hiding in one of the lounges with her books. Tom never stopped talking except to whistle and was thereby the source of universal irritation; he was also nearly six foot tall but, when we had to work in pairs, always let his partner take most of the weight and do most of the work. Jon flirted, or tried to, with everyone and was something of a creep; meeting me once on the stairs, he bodily picked me up and swung me round in an oppressive bear hug while I shouted at him to stop. Mary was the sanest, most sensible person in the place and loved by everyone;

half-jokingly, half-seriously, we called her 'Matron', because she wore the uniform dress instead of the tunic, cinched neatly at the waist with a wide elastic belt. Sheryl, she who gave me the Shakespeare, called me Mary Poppins because of my long blue coat, my red heeled shoes and, she said, "The way you hold your lunch bag when you ring the doorbell in the morning." Hannah, James, Mary, Celine; Marge, Leila, Chelsea, Lynn: a kaleidoscope of human nature, always shifting and changing, altering constantly around a small coterie of immutables. War, they say, makes for strange bedfellows. So did Covid.

5

VARIETY IS THE SPICE OF LIFE

The title of this chapter is, in case you didn't pick up on the heavily dripping sarcasm, ironic. The daily institutionalised regime of a care home offers little scope for variety, and there was none at all during the strange, surreal, dystopian lockdowns, when hours and shifts and days blurred together, and time became almost meaningless. Locked away in our hermetically sealed prison, only the television programmes marked the passing of the days and reminded us that there was still a world beyond the care home walls. *Eggheads* on Mondays. *Vera* on Thursdays. *Songs of Praise* on Sundays. In that first, longest, hardest lockdown, it was weeks before the residents were allowed out of their rooms. It was many more weeks before Barbara, the activities lady, was allowed back in to do her job. It was months before visitors were allowed, under the most unnatural circumstances: gloved, gowned, masked, ushered by the external door into the broiling hot conservatory, separated from their mother or father by the closed glass door, forced to communicate by shouting into an intermittently working intercom system. Even as the rest of the country inched towards a 'new normal' (hateful phrase!), normality remained very far away for care homes and their residents. I sometimes wonder if, in some homes, it will ever return. Even if it does, it will be far too late for many. For each resident who died of or with Covid, there are several more who survived but whose decline has been irreversibly hastened. They have forgotten how to wash, feed and toilet themselves, or now exist sunk into a stuporous and unrousable depression. Some of them, separated for so long, will never again recognise their families and friends. Not the lockdowns, not the restrictions, could prevent Covid from entering care homes, but the suffering they caused was catastrophic.

Get people up. Get them washed and dressed. Breakfast. Clear breakfast. Morning tea. Toileting. Lunch. Clear lunch. Afternoon tea. Toileting. Supper. Clear supper. Bed. This was the unchanging skeleton on which every day hung. In theory, of course, every resident was supposed to do what they liked, when they liked, and of course this was impossible. Despite the lip service we tried to pay to the 'person-centred approach', an institution cannot be run without a routine. The monotony nearly drove me mad, but it was infinitely worse for the residents. In the colder weather, for months on end, often they did not even put a nose outdoors, not even into the little courtyard garden.

Each day was entirely predictable. Also entirely predictable was the impossibility of doing our job properly. We did not spend our shifts as relatives fondly – or foolishly

– thought we did: sitting with the residents, holding hands, talking, reading, laughing, walking peacefully round the garden to smell the roses. Those adverts you see, of a care worker helping an immaculately made up elderly lady with a jigsaw, one arm lovingly draped around her shoulder, no mask nor PPE in sight, beaming smiles plastered across both faces? They weren't made by anyone with experience of working in care. We spent shifts running from one task to the next, always behind, always stressed, always hot, someone always wanting to know why no. 37 wasn't up yet and why no. 9 had no. 26's trousers on, and where were no. 8's hearing aids, and could you hurry up with the hoist in no. 6's room because it was needed in no. 10's, and why wasn't no. 13 coming down for breakfast, and oh, here was a senior to ask did we know it was nearly 10am, and why wasn't the dining room cleared yet? Our smiles, I am afraid, were scarce.

Some smug idiot way beyond us, way beyond even Lynn, and certainly way beyond the practical realities of actually working with the elderly, had apparently worked out that fifteen minutes was sufficient for helping a resident up in the morning to get ready for the day. On a full corridor of ten residents, that meant two and half hours to get everyone up, so if we came on shift at 7am every resident should, in theory, have got to the dining room by 9:30am. This was where that magic deadline originated. It was never met, even though the night staff always started getting people up before the day staff started. Think about it: fifteen minutes to coax someone out of bed, give them a shower or full body wash, shave them, apply creams, find clothes for the day, having first asked them what they want to wear, brush hair, clean spectacles, check and insert hearing aids, clean and fit dentures, strip soiled bedlinen, sort and bag the washing, complete the paperwork. Remember that the person you are assisting is of, at best, limited mobility and not infrequently bed-bound; that they may refuse to get up; they may resist you at every turn; they may be verbally or physically aggressive. Fifteen minutes? Impossible.

We all hated the time constraints, but they were especially resented by some of the older carers, who remembered working in care in the days when it was less about box-ticking and more about actually caring. Andrea remained unmoved by imposed pressures of time and doggedly insisted on giving each resident the time she thought they needed. Laudable, of course, except that there was simply never enough time, and someone else would end up having to pick up some of her work, causing annoyance and resentment. The balance was an impossible one.

There was just one time of the day where things were sometimes quiet enough to spend 'quality time' (how I hate that phrase) with residents. This was the first hour of the afternoon shift, as long as you weren't on tea-trolley duty. Replete from lunch and not yet needing the toilet pre-tea, most residents spent this time gently snoozing in the lounges. I would go to find little Georgina, prise her away from Ethel's side and take her off for a shower. Yes, 2:30pm is a strange time for a shower, but it was the only time to do it properly, making it leisurely and enjoyable instead of a stressful flurry. Afterwards, I would sit her down in the tiny room always called the 'salon' – where I had been interviewed that March day so long ago – and set her hair in rollers. I had always been good at hair, a legacy from my ballet dancing days, but never in my ballet days had I used rollers, assuming vaguely that they had been left behind with World War II. It took me a while to get the hang of them, but Georgina always seemed delighted with the results, though to begin with the fact that she had very bad eyesight may have been fortunate. But I would tell her she looked beautiful, and she would squeeze my hand and giggle like a girl, and for a brief moment, I would feel pride in my work instead of resentful dread.

Shifts, when I started at Ember Vale at the height of the pandemic's first wave, were twelve hours long, an emergency situation designed partly to reduce the number of staff coming into the building each day and partly in response to many staff being off sick or forced to isolate. It was weeks before the normal shift pattern resumed: the early (7am–2:20pm), the late (2pm–9:20pm) and the night shift (9pm–7:20am). Even then, staff shortages meant that double shifts, from 8am to 8pm, occasionally popped up on our rosters unbidden (some staff preferred the twelve-hour shifts, or 'long days', and kept on this pattern after the rest of us had thankfully gone back to mere seven-hour days). There was a period when, even more understaffed than usual, fourteen-hour days started mysteriously appearing. These came to a swift end when we discovered that, despite working from 7am to past 9pm, we were only paid for twelve hours; the other two, apparently, were classed as legally required 'rest hours' and therefore not eligible for pay. There was outrage among the staff and Lynn, wisely, quietly dropped these shifts. Not that she had much choice, for we simply refused to work them.

We were supposed to have every other weekend off, which never, ever happened. Often, I worked six in a row. Staff on full-time hours often did eight. At least once a week, we had back-to-back shifts: rostered on for the late one night and the early the following morning, a pattern which breaches an employee's right to eleven hours' rest between working days. Friday night/Saturday morning back-to-backs were the most depressing way possible to start a weekend, but in the middle of morning sickness, I was rostered on for three back-to-backs within a week. It just about finished me off.

Handovers began each shift, at least to begin with. All the staff coming on duty would crowd into the office with the senior coming off duty, and we would sit down with cups of tea and sheets of paper purloined from the printer to take down any necessary notes on each resident. It was an efficient and effective way of making sure that everyone was on the same page and that nothing got missed. Then the powers that be decided that having everyone squashed into the office couldn't possibly continue as it breached social distancing, and we were all made to join a WhatsApp group where the handover notes were sent to our phones. So instead of everyone crowding into the office with cups of tea to hear handover, everyone crowded into the staff room with cups of tea to read it. This, apparently, was progress. It was unpopular: information got missed or left out; the handover message was frequently sent late, and we would then be in trouble for not being on the floor; and the messages came relentlessly, three times a day, whether or not you were actually at work. We complained, but to no avail. Leila refused to have work messages on her phone and, whenever readded to the group by an irate senior, simply removed herself again. I would look on in envy and wish I had her chutzpah.

The first tentative rearrangement of lockdown restrictions in the outside world brought no change for care home staff. We still had to be swaddled in plastic PPE within an inch of our lives, suffocating in masks, gloves and aprons, sitting an impossible two metres apart in the tiny staff room on breaks. But with upper management heralding a 'new normal' (hateful phrase!), the residents were finally allowed out of their bedrooms to a slightly expanded incarceration. In their wisdom, management had decreed that residents should mix only in small preordained groups; sensible in theory, perhaps, but impossible to put into practice. Lynn did what she usually did when faced with an impossible order from on high, which was to try to make it work, shout at us all for a week while we failed miserably to make it work, then quietly abandon it when it became abundantly clear that it couldn't possibly work. So the residents were divided into five groups; each group was allocated one of the five lounges; and there the residents had to stay, all day long, from getting up to going to bed. Two metres apart. At all times.

Of course it didn't work. To begin with, the lounges were small and cramped; Lynn gamely engaged in some very creative measuring, eventually succeeding in convincing herself that all the chairs were dutifully situated two metres from each other. They weren't. Then – not unreasonably, given they had spent weeks deprived of almost all human contact – it proved impossible to explain to the residents a.) that they had to keep apart and b.) why. I came in once to find two little old ladies – fast friends before the lockdown and still, semi-miraculously, able to recognise each other and their friendship – sitting companionably in the same big armchair, comparing invisible knitting stitches and wondering earnestly how long rationing was going to last. They were the happiest they had been in weeks. But Lynn's thundering footsteps were advancing down the corridor, and so, sighing, I tried to separate them. This was met with a duet of polite refusals.

"Oh, no, dear, I couldn't leave my friend!"

"It's much warmer here, dear, than in that chair." (This in a room where the thermostat never dipped below 25°C.)

I gave up and left them to it. Lynn marched in and told me off. I told her to try and stamped off, scowling, to the staff toilet, where I hid on occasions where everything was getting too much. As my sentence at Ember Vale wore on, I spent more and more time in this retreat. Never for long, five or ten minutes at a time, but in order to preserve what remained of my sanity I had to, had to be alone, had to shut the door against the cares and jobs and recriminations that pressed so hard from every side there was no room to breathe. Come to think of it, now that I have children, I still do exactly this. I dump them both in their cots, lock myself in the bathroom and, with a sigh of relief, sit down to pee in peace.

Most of the residents did not get on so well as the companions in the armchair. Fights and altercations were frequent, sometimes turning physical. These were most commonly about seating arrangements ("That's my chair!" Well, no, you might usually sit there, but it's not actually *yours*; you can't stop Jack from sitting on it), sometimes about possessions ("That's my newspaper!" Well, no, it's from the communal library and anyway, it's two years old), occasionally about desire ("That's my wife!" No, she's definitely not, and *please*, you really can't take your pants down in the middle of the corridor). Sometimes there were personality clashes; Cindy and Marion clashed with every single resident (and each other) as well as every single member of staff. But whereas the staff had to remain professional, the residents, released from propriety by their lack of capacity, were free to scratch, spit and hiss like fighting cats. This some of them did. But most of the time, slumped in armchairs, stewing in the tropical heat of the lounges, most of them merely slept or dozed, a cacophony of snores, wheezes, gurgles and coughs competing with the blare of the telly. Each of them sitting in the same lounge, in the same chair, day after day, month after month, year after year if they lived that long.

The home's activities coordinator, Barbara, struggled valiantly to introduce some stimulation into the daily monotony. There was bingo; there were quizzes; there was a book club after lunch; there were arts and crafts tailored to high days and holidays like Easter, Christmas and Valentine's Day. But even these became repetitive and stale, and Barbara's soft, gentle voice reading in the overwarm lounge would merely lull her audience back to noisy sleep.

Fourteen months after the beginning of the first lockdown, there was great excitement when Lynn gave permission for a select group of half a dozen residents to issue forth for their first outside trip in all those months. This was an operation which makes getting out of the house with two under-twos, a procedure which is now wont to leave me faint and exhausted, look like a piece of cake. I passed a harassed Barbara in the corridor, struggling with wheelchairs and walkers and a bag stuffed with continence aids and spare clothes, and envied her not at all, even though outside the bright sunshine called temptingly.

Normally, there was eager competition to run the errands which took us off the premises. Usually, these errands were to one of the local pharmacies or doctor's surgeries, to pick up medication or drop off specimens, or else to the Co-op which stood across the road from the home, to buy fags either for Gwyneth (eighty-three and an inveterate chain smoker) or the senior on duty (most of whom were also inveterate smokers at work despite the fact that this was a sackable offence). One of these errands was the first, and so far only, occasion on which I bought a packet of cigarettes; I had to ask the senior who sent me to write down what she wanted. In I trotted and put the piece of paper down on the till, still wearing my carer's tunic and conscious that this was not exactly a good look. The boy behind the till did not even try to hide his smirk.

I preferred being sent to the pharmacy or surgery, and these runs fairly often fell to me because I had a car; several of the staff did not drive and were completely reliant either on public transport, their own two legs or lifts from colleagues. Of course I was never offered reimbursement for the petrol; oh dear no, of course not. But I was glad to go anyway, to speed along country lanes with the windows open to blow away the care home smell and the radio blaring to drown out the care home noise still ringing in my head.

One day about a month before Christmas, Barbara collared me in the corridor. All conversations of any importance seemed to take place in the corridors, despite the fact that this was frowned upon by the seniors and by Lynn. These liminal spaces, places of transience through which we endlessly hurried, nevertheless functioned as the spaces in which we met and were briefly held together before being dispersed again upon the waters of chaos.

Barbara said to me now: "You used to be in musical theatre, didn't you?"

This myth had somehow spread unbidden through the home. I never spoke of my pre-Covid life, so where it came from I have no idea. In any case, like most myths, once it had sprung into life, it proved impossible to kill.

No, I had never taken part in musical theatre. The idea of singing, in public, on stage, was a terrifying one. For me and for the audience.

"But you used to act, didn't you?" pressed Barbara.

No, I didn't do that either. But she persisted, so I tried to explain that I had studied theatre, worked in theatre, directed theatre, choreographed theatre, written about theatre, run theatre both front of house and back of house, in fact been involved with theatre in just about any aspect except acting or, heaven forbid, singing.

This was met with the blank look with which it was always met. I really should have known better. So, instead, I said: "Why do you ask?"

She explained that, in normal times, the home organised a trip to the pantomime every Christmas. This, obviously, was off the cards that year. But she had an idea. The home could put on its own nativity play, produced and performed by the staff under her direction.

I considered this a brave and noble and extremely rash idea, but did not have the heart to tell her so. Instead, I promised to give her support both moral and practical as long as it did not involve acting nor, under any circumstances, singing. So she press-ganged a recalcitrant troupe of actors and became more and more harassed. But Barbara possessed the two qualities essential in any director: she coped stoically with her cast as they bickered, squabbled, giggled, lost their scripts, failed to learn their lines, failed to attend rehearsals and dropped out completely at the last minute; and she was remarkably good at getting people to do things they didn't want to do. This was how I ended up, two days before Christmas, narrating what was probably the least-rehearsed nativity play in production history.

As a performance it was dreadful. Everybody read off the scripts, having completely neglected to learn the lines in time; nobody could speak clearly, let alone project, because we were not allowed to remove our masks; one of the three wise men had been recruited at the eleventh hour after her predecessor failed to turn up for the shift that day; the carols dragged appallingly and were completely out of tune. And yet – and yet – it somehow caught the essential magic of theatre: the power to bring people together and transport them out of time and space, beyond self, suffering and boredom. It was the worst performance I have ever seen, and the most moving. There we were, locked in the home, all theatres across the land closed and all festive activities banned, our audience abandoned and alone, and still the natural human instinct to seek solace in creative expression flourished.

By working the late shift Christmas Eve and again on Boxing Day, I managed to get Christmas Day itself off. Those who worked the bank holidays received no extra pay for doing so. Previously, they had been entitled to double pay, but just before I started, dear NG had removed this. It was a strange and sombre Christmas; usually Barbara would swamp the home with elves and gnomes, Santas and reindeer, festoons of lights and several Christmas trees and goodness knows what else. But that year, in case the virus lurked in the baubles, the Covid grinches ding donging tinnily on high allowed us only one sparsely decorated tree. By 8pm on Christmas Eve, most of the residents were already in bed; a few sat on in the main lounge, and there we congregated in the undecorated gloom, the carol service from King's College Cambridge tinkling out from the telly. The camaraderie and jollity of the nativity play the day before had already dissipated. Everyone was simply waiting for the shift to end, wanting to get home to children and family and their own cosily decorated homes. We congregated round the table, in flagrant breach of the two-metre rule, and sat down, hoping to get the paperwork completed in time for a swift getaway at 9:20pm.

But lo, here entered the senior, brandishing tambourines and maracas!

I blinked. Had the anticipatory stiff gin with which David usually greeted me after a late shift started working in advance?

No, we had to perform an impromptu carol concert, to be filmed by the senior and uploaded to the home's Facebook page so that the residents' families could see what a merry Christmas their loved ones were having. Somewhere on the internet there exists video footage of a forlorn group of carers performing a raggedy rendition of 'Jingle Bells'. As its half-hearted strains petered out, the radio, on in competition with the telly, struck up 'Have Yourself a Merry Little Christmas', the song that for the month of December had replaced 'We'll Meet Again' as the most played song on air.

It was my first Christmas away from home. It would be years before the fates, or God, or Covid, allowed us all to be together again.

On Boxing Day morning, at an early hour when most people were either still fast asleep or, blearily remembering the festivities of the day before, nursing regrets of varying kinds, we were woken by a bluish light filtering through the grey gloom of pre-dawn and making kaleidoscopic patterns on the bedroom ceiling. I peered round the edge of the curtain. An ambulance was parked outside the house, and coming from downstairs were movements and voices I did not recognise.

"They've called an ambulance," I reported in alarm to David.

His father had been 'under the weather' for a few weeks – tired, coughing, a bit breathless. But overnight, his breathing had become much worse, and with it, he had developed bad chest pain. Getting a GP appointment was impossible. The NHS 111 phone line was, as ever, 'experiencing an extremely high volume of callers at present'. Not knowing what else to do, David's sister had called 999. The fact that they sent an immediate response, at a time of critical national shortage when care home residents regularly waited eight hours or more for an ambulance, was not reassuring. How bad must he be, if they would actually send an ambulance?

The paramedics thought he was in heart failure. In the darkness, he was driven off to hospital, his family left behind to wait and worry. All that morning, we heard nothing. I went to work, surreptitiously checking my phone whenever I could. No news. No news by the time I got home at 10pm that night, only faces etched with worry and strain and a tense silence pervading the normally busy house. No news the next morning. I rang the hospital switchboard, spending an hour on hold, then half an hour more being passed between wards and departments. Finally, a nurse came on the line and confirmed that yes, my father-in-law was on her ward, and yes, it was heart failure, an arrhythmia caused by atrial fibrillation. Clearly used to panicking relations responding with horror to these long and dire-sounding words, she then said calmly, "But it's not a death sentence, you know." Relief made my thanks effusive, relief due not only to her words but also to having finally got through to a real person who could utter them. Yes, she went on, still calmly, he could have a visitor, but only one, and they could only come at one particular hour, for fifteen minutes only, and they would have to wear full PPE. Oh, and they would not actually be allowed on the ward; they could communicate only through its glass doors, no touching or handholding or hugging permitted. Then she was gone, back to her never-ending round of duties, or on to the next relative frantic for news.

This encounter with a dystopian NHS had for us a happy ending. Medication brought the arrhythmia under control and, in a few days, one lucky patient was released back to a very relieved family. For other families, other encounters and other endings were not happy. The cancellation of all treatment, procedures and operations other than those related to Covid had an immediate and devastating effect.

Words, stories, grief, anger, incomprehension, disbelief: swirling through the corridors, swapped in the office, permeating the staff room.

Myrtle's cataract operation cancelled. Myrtle therefore going blind within a few weeks. Justine's sister's cancer treatment, to which she had been responding well, cancelled. Justine's sister therefore dead by Christmas. Doris's appointment for new dentures cancelled. Doris therefore obliged to eat nothing but mush. Gwyneth's hip replacement cancelled. Gwyneth therefore confined to a wheelchair for the rest of her shortened days. And this only at one mid-size care home – one tiny little community. What devastation was mirrored and replicated across the country? What other lives were lost or blighted, what anger goes unexpressed, what grief unacknowledged? By the media and politicians much was made, that first, longest lockdown, of invoking the British spirit of the Blitz, Vera Lynn the soundtrack to those long, weary days. Every parish in the country has its memorial to those killed in war. Will there one day be memorials to those killed or maimed by lockdown? Will they too have their names inscribed in gold and underneath the words, *Never Again*?

6

BLOOD, TOIL, TEARS AND SHIT

It lay in the middle of the worn carpet, a neat sausage turd, inordinately large. A trail of smaller blobs, gleaming strangely pale like the pebbles of Hansel and Gretel, led down the corridor beyond to a bedroom door. I knew which bedroom door they disappeared behind. I knew who had pale stools (the result of a liver problem) and who had black stools (the result of iron supplements). I knew who produced pebbles and who produced sausages, whose stools were always runny and who was chronically constipated. The Bristol Stool Chart, which hung on the back of every bathroom door with its graphic little illustrative diagrams and strangely poetic text, was our catechism. *Type 1 – separate hard lumps, like nuts (hard to pass). Type 2 – sausage-shaped but lumpy. Type 3 – like a sausage but with cracks on its surface. Type 4 – like a sausage or snake, smooth and soft. Type 5 – soft blobs with clear-cut edges (passed easily). Type 6 – Fluffy pieces with ragged edges, a mushy stool. Type 7 – watery, no solid pieces. Entirely liquid.*

We all feared this last, the dreaded 'loose bowels', which precipitated immediate isolation for the unfortunate sufferer. It is a strange and bizarre world to work in, one where you can immediately identify someone by their stools. We knew them so well, the residents – and yet we hardly knew them at all. We knew every detail of their most intimate bodily functions and almost nothing at all about the people they had been, the lives they had lived, before dementia came stealing in, before they entered the home.

There is definitely a 'care home look', which, with its uniformity and blandness, further erodes individuality. Everyone looks the same, and it is so easy to forget that everyone is so very different. Although a couple of the women had wardrobes, drawers and cupboards stuffed to overflowing, many of the residents seemed to enter with pitifully few possessions, and of those most were clothes (though very few had enough underwear). Family photographs were surprisingly sparse; few had many knick-knacks and ornaments; fewer still had any books. And the clothes were all the same, irrespective of which wardrobe you looked into: knickers or underwear (full briefs) from Marks and Spencer; outer clothes (loose skirts for the women, grungy tracksuit bottoms for the men, baggy T-shirts for both) from Peacocks. Easier to dress in, of course, when you have stiff limbs or limited mobility, but I did sometimes yearn for a modicum of style. And colour: drab darks predominated. Gwyneth had a cotton jersey top, very simple in cut and shape but a gorgeous sunflower yellow. I used to offer this top more than any other just for the spark of colour it provided amidst the general gloom.

There is a story, possibly apocryphal, that sales of red lipstick went up during the Blitz. Women wore it to give themselves courage, project confidence and stick a finger up at Hitler. Of the residents, only Ethel ever wore make-up, but she carefully applied it every day, always finishing with a swipe of bright-red lipstick. Some of the carers wore lipstick too, every shift behind their masks, sticking the finger up at Covid.

The predominant colour of the care home, however, was beige – or perhaps brown. The days were beige, and the shit was brown. Several of my most prominent memories of Ember Vale seem to revolve around faeces. There was the incident of the poo pebbles, and there was the time a resident on end-of-life care lashed out while being given continence care, smearing excrement all over Mary's face, arms, apron and tunic, and there was the time, coming on to the morning shift, I met one of the night staff popping out of a bedroom, doing her last rounds before going off shift.

"You just come on?" she said. "Good luck." And she laughed and went home.

I put my head round the door. The room was smeared with faeces. It was on the bedding, the bed, the walls, the floor; along with a handful of paper towels, it had clogged the sink, which, the tap having been left running, was now overflowing; it was on the seat, arms and legs of the commode; in short, it was everywhere, except actually *in* the commode. It did not seem possible that so much could come out of one person. The smell was abominable.

There was one upside to dealing with this. No nappy my children can produce has the power to horrify me.

We dealt with urine too, of course; there was one occasion where the front foyer was turned into a slippery skating rink by a gentleman who decided the floor needed watering. And, on a lesser scale, we encountered various other bodily fluids, mostly vomit and blood. I remember Martin, vomiting his life away. And Gladys, admitted to hospital as a day patient for a colonoscopy. She came back very quiet, was installed in a chair in the lounge, and, amid the usual busyness of a shift, was promptly left to her own devices. Rushing into the room on another errand entirely, I spied a pool of some darkish liquid underneath her chair. I thought at first it was tea but, rushing back with mop and wet floor sign, was horrified to realise it was in fact blood. It was literally dripping from her, running down the back of the chair and pooling underneath, but she seemed completely unaware. In fact, she was probably, not unreasonably, in shock.

I rushed to get the senior. The senior rushed to call 999, who told her to call 111, who as usual were 'experiencing a very high volume of calls at present'. I mopped up the blood, put a towel underneath the chair to catch what was still dripping down, made Gladys a mug of sweet tea and went back to whatever I had been doing before.

Scurrying by the office half an hour later, the senior called me in. Thrusting the telephone at me, she said, "They have to speak to you because you found it."

Unwillingly, I took the phone. A young, brusque male voice snapped questions on the other end of the line.

"Am I speaking with the person who found the, um, fluid?"

"Yes."

"Name?"

"Eleanor Bloomfield."

"Position?"

"Care Assistant."

"Name of person on whose behalf you are speaking?"

"Gladys Bakewell."

"Date of birth?"

"Hasn't the senior already told you all this?"

"We need it from you."

The senior had left Gladys's file open on the desk and I flipped frantically through it while the call handler tutted on the other end of the line. We were supposed to know the details and medical history of each resident, but with forty to memorise, at least half of whom changed on a regular basis, it was impossible. Eventually, I found her date of birth.

"The 2nd of July 1936."

"NHS number?"

More frantic fumbling. I found it at last.

"Medical history?"

More fumbling. "Um, Gladys is living with vascular dementia... she was admitted today for a scheduled colonoscopy to investigate suspected—"

But he wasn't really interested. "Please describe why you are calling."

"Surely the senior—?"

"We need it from you."

"Well, Gladys is bleeding, rectally I think."

"How do you know it's blood?"

"Pardon?"

"How do you know it's blood?"

"I know what blood looks like!"

"How do you know it's rectal bleeding?"

"She had a colonoscopy earlier today."

"How much fluid, er, blood is there?"

I panicked slightly. At the best of times, I struggle with numbers and with estimating size, volume or amounts. As I hesitated, he impatiently spoke again. "Bigger than a 50p piece?"

"Yes, definitely."

"More than two hundred millilitres?"

I tried to imagine whether that dark, sinister pool would fill one of the mugs we served tea in. The mugs held two hundred and fifty millilitres. "Yes, I think so."

"You think?"

"Yes."

"Well, can't you go and measure it?"

"No."

"Why not?"

"Because I wiped it up."

"Why did you do that?"

"Because she was bleeding all over the floor!"

Speaking very slowly and clearly, "Well, I need to know the *exact* amount. You don't seem to understand. You aren't being very helpful…"

I lost it. "Look. I may be a care assistant, but *I am not stupid*!" And I thrust the phone back at the astonished senior and stormed out. I am not proud of this.

I went back to Gladys, whose corner of the lounge now resembled a scene from *Macbeth*. Eventually, the bleeding did stop, and in a day or two, she seemed to recover. This was lucky, because 111 refused to send anyone out or have her seen. "Just observe and call us back if it gets worse." For all they knew or cared, Gladys could have haemorrhaged to death.

From beginning to end of a shift, we toiled unceasingly, even if it was a 'quiet' shift without any bodily fluids out of the ordinary. Sitting on the beds was strictly verboten but often, having helped someone onto the commode and while waiting for them to finish, we did sit, just for a few minutes, just to take the weight off our feet. No, it wasn't professional. But we were so tired.

These moments of random stillness sometimes led to odd moments of connection: between carer and carer, and between carers and resident. One day, working with Chelsea for the pre-lunch doubles toileting rounds, we came to Maisie's room. I knocked and in we trailed with the rotunda, banging it as always against the doorframe and removing a few more flakes of paint. Chelsea pushed the rotunda up against the chair, helping Maisie to plant her feet in the middle of the rotating base and grip the handles. I found the control for the recliner armchair and raised the chair, slowly tipping it up and forward so that Maisie was helped to a semi-standing position. Then I put one hand on Maisie's back to steady her; Chelsea released the catch on the rotunda and turned the base through ninety degrees; and in one fluid movement, I slid the commode in behind Maisie with one hand and pulled her trousers down with the other. It was a choreographed dance we had all performed together many times before.

"You can sit down now, darlin'," Chelsea said. "Do you want us to stay or give you a minute?"

Maisie grunted. "Stay. Won't be long."

Chelsea and I flopped down to sit on the bed. Chelsea groaned. "Ooooh, me feet!"

I gazed out of the window. Always, whenever I had half a chance, I did this, in search of an existence beyond the care home walls. It was midwinter: grey trees stood stark against a grey sky. Moving across the general grey was a scurrying blob of darker grey fur.

I pointed. "Look. Squirrel!"

Chelsea gave me an odd look. "You are funny, Eleanor. Why do you care about an old squirrel?"

"Because we're in here, and it's out there."

Now Chelsea pointed too. "Look, Maisie. Squirrel."

And all three of us – resident on the commode, carers on the bed – sat and looked out of the window at a grey squirrel running free through the bare winter trees.

Maisie was so sparrow-thin that one of us could easily have helped her onto the commode alone. But it was a strict regulation that using the rotunda had to be done in pairs. Like every other regulation, this was often ignored under duress. Short on time and short on staff, some of the carers would occasionally quietly go solo with the residents who were light enough. Many of them were. Often stick-thin to begin with, almost all new residents entering a care home will lose weight. At Ember Vale all residents were weighed once a month, and those who had lost weight since the previous measurement were put on a food and fluid chart. On this was supposed to be recorded everything the resident ate or drank over the course of a day and how much. It was probably the most hated piece of paperwork in the entire place.

It sounds simple in theory and completely laudable. In practice it was a complete nightmare. No foolproof way of completing the charts was ever found and responsibility for them changed continuously. Sometimes each carer was responsible for the charts of the residents on their own corridor; sometimes one carer alone, the float, was designated responsible for *all* the charts. Completing them accurately was next to impossible. Oh, it sounds simple enough. But three-quarters of the home was on a food and fluid chart; keeping track of what thirty different people – spread across lounges, dining room and bedrooms – are eating and drinking, remembering it all and entering it into the charts – which, for data protection reasons, we were not allowed to carry with us; they had to be locked into the record room unless we were actually completing them – all while trying to do all the other jobs and attend to all the myriad minor emergencies of a typical shift – is much more difficult than it sounds.

Even worse than trying to complete the paperwork was the anxiety of trying to ensure the residents actually consumed food and fluid to be recorded. The elderly often eat very little. The elderly in care homes often eat particularly little. The noise, the bustle, the regimented mealtimes, the lack of physical activity, the prevalence of anxiety and depression, the unappetising food – all are not conducive to hearty appetites. But if residents failed to meet the targets for nutritional intake, or regain weight lost, there was all hell to pay, because the home would be required to inform the GP, and this would reflect badly in an inspection.

You can't force someone to eat and drink. But it seemed that this was exactly what we were expected to do. Lynn was not remotely interested in protestations that we had tried, we really had, to persuade Maisie and Martin to eat dinner and drink a cup of tea, *but they just didn't want to.* As long as the paperwork showed sufficient intake, that was all that mattered. And when it didn't, God help us.

I think this is why I now intensely dislike feeding my toddler. I hate attempting to spoon food into a reluctant mouth only to have it refused. I feel guilty if he won't eat yet lack time and patience for endless coaxing and distracting. I keep a mental tally of all that he has consumed and worry that it is insufficient. Somewhere in the back of my head, along with the bells that still need answering and the paperwork that still needs completing, is a food and fluid chart that still needs recording.

Any parent of toddlers will tell you that life is all downhill after 4pm. The day dissolves into an ever-descending spiral of boredom, hunger, tears and tantrums, only brought to a close by the blessed hour of Bedtime. So too is there an extended witching hour in care homes. After tea is served, and before residents start going to bed, there is a natural slump in the rhythm of the day. Manager, receptionist and activities staff have left; the domestic staff will shortly be going off shift and are killing time until they do; visitors have gone home, shooed away before tea ("we find our residents eat better without distraction"); the kitchen staff are winding down for the day. The telephone, for the first time since 8am, is allowed breathing space, for medical administrative staff – ringing continuously throughout the day to arrange, rearrange or cancel appointments, follow-ups or test results – do not work past 5:30pm. Only the carers are left, reluctantly facing the long slog of evening before they too finally get to leave. And it is at this point that all hell breaks loose.

There were more recordable incidents – falls (so many falls), outbursts of aggression or violence, attempted escapes ("I've *got* to go home, *now*, before bedtime"), or simply

Gregory deciding to rearrange the bathroom plumbing – at this point of early evening than at any other time of day. Nobody was quite sure why. Lynn became convinced it was lack of stimulation and persuaded Barbara to trial some evening activities. It made no difference.

The falls were the most common problem. In my humble opinion, based on observation and experience, residents were more likely to fall in the evening because they were most tired then. But a high falls rate looks bad in an inspection report, and so Lynn decreed that the falls rate had to come down. Since she could hardly prevent the residents from being tired in the evenings, and since there were not enough staff to monitor all the residents properly and forestall any untoward incidents, those judged most at risk of falling were subjected to a seat sensor. This was a pad placed on the seat of a chair; when the occupant stood up, an alarm was sent either to the call bell system or, later, in what was hailed as progress, to an alarm box carried by a designated carer in the pocket of her tunic. The sensitivity levels varied wildly. Sometimes the sensor went off as a resident slumbered peacefully in the chair; sometimes we would find a resident vaguely wandering the corridors, the sensor having completely failed to activate when they got up.

The home had only three seat sensors so, as the falls rate remained stubbornly stable, other residents classed as high risk were monitored with a PIR (passive infrared) sensor. These detected any movement within range, so if a resident did not actually stand up but merely moved an arm or a leg, or if a carer or domestic walked in front it, not realising it was there, the sensor would go off regardless. The result was that we were continually running backwards and forwards to reset the sensors, and the effect on the falls rate was precisely zero. It became ridiculous: sometimes we did nothing but reset sensors, especially if the resident was confined to their bedroom in isolation. There were two dreadful days when Gregory, in isolation following a hospital visit – and whose bedroom was upstairs, in the furthest reaches of the building, equidistant from stairs and lift – had a PIR sensor after a near-miss fall. Normally, Gregory's mobility was quite reasonable; he used a wheeled walker, but generally he was perfectly steady and pottered around without concern. The near-miss was an anomaly. Nevertheless, there had been a recent rash of falls, to which Lynn's knee-jerk reaction was to increase the number of residents monitored with sensors. So a sensor Gregory had to have.

We tried to explain to him that he had to stay sitting in his chair. Of course he couldn't understand why, and of course he kept getting up. That morning, I did nothing but run backwards and forwards to turn off the sensor and reset it. Often, it would go off again before I had reached the stairs. Sometimes it went off before I was even out of the room. At last, in maddened despair, I turned the wretched thing off.

But alas, the senior on duty that morning was Lucy. Lucy possessed an almost obsessive compulsion for doing things by the book. (She was the only person in the entire home who consistently, without fail, followed the tortuous multiple-step process for donning and doffing PPE. She then wondered why she was always behind with her work and never left a shift on time.) This was, in a way, admirable, but she completely lacked common sense. She also lacked any tact and was continually popping up at shoulder or elbow to berate us for some overlook or omission. Even Lynn thought she took it a bit too far. Finally, she had an immaculate pixie haircut with blonde highlights – the kind of style that grows out very quickly and needs continual maintenance to keep its shape and colour. Lucy's hairstyle never altered, never, not once, not through all the lockdowns when hairdresser's appointments were supposedly banned. Either it was a wig, or Lucy (or a member of her household) was very, very good at DIY hairdressing, or, outside of work, Lucy was not quite so scrupulous at rule-following as she pretended to be, and quietly visited a hairdresser operating, equally quietly, underground.

But we were at work, and by some evil fate, Lucy managed to materialise at my shoulder just as I emerged from Gregory's room. Damn. Caught.

"What are you doing?" she asked.

"Turning off the sensor."

"Turning *off* the sensor?" she queried, raising perfectly arched eyebrows beneath that maddeningly perfect pixie haircut.

"Yes."

"Don't you know that Lynn has given instructions that this resident is to be on a sensor?"

"Yes."

When she caught us in some failing, Lucy liked to adopt a tone more in sorrow than in anger. "So why did you turn it off?"

"Because he keeps getting up; I keep having to turn it off; I can't get any work done; and he doesn't need a sensor anyway."

Sorrowfully, Lucy shook that pixie-cropped head. "But Lynn has said he has to be on a sensor."

"Well, you answer it then. Or tell Lynn to."

"That is not my job."

Stand-off. Eventually, muttering darkly, I yielded and turned the wretched thing back on, then stalked down the corridor with Lucy wafting behind. The sensor went off again as we reached the lift. The doors opened just as I got there and Chelsea, my doubles toileting partner, appeared. She was very cross.

"Where the *hell* have you been?"

"Sensor."

"Well, hurry up, we're well behind."

Down we went, leaving Lucy on the landing mouthing something about a sensor needing to be attended to. As the lift shuddered and groaned its way downwards, Chelsea said, "Why didn't you just turn the bloody thing off?"

"I tried to."

"*She* catch you?"

"Yup."

The sensors were, for us, intensely annoying, but no worse than that. For the residents, they meant a serious loss of liberty, independence and dignity. (Imagine how you would feel, if, every time you tried to stand up, a carer popped up and shouted at you, "Sit down, darlin', *sit down!*") Yet, unforgivably, the CQC's paranoia around the falls rate meant that some residents never walked again. It was as simple as that.

One day Doris arrived, living with mid-stage dementia but fully independently mobile. While incarcerated in her room for the two-week isolation period, she fell; nobody was quite sure how or why. She had no previous history of falls.

Nevertheless, social services insisted that she use a Zimmer frame, 'to reduce the risk of further falls'. Once she was allowed out of her room, we were constantly running after her: "You forgot your frame, Doris!" She never got the hang of using it. One wheel squeaked dreadfully (why didn't we ask the maintenance man to oil it, I wonder now?) and to avoid this, she drove the frame on one edge, lifting two of the four wheels clean off the floor. One afternoon just after tea, heading back from dining room to lounge, she caught the raised edge of the frame on the door post and fell crashing to the floor. Lynn, backed up by social services, insisted she now use a seat sensor and not walk anywhere unsupervised. But they needn't have bothered, for with this second fall, Doris had lost all her confidence, and she refused to walk anywhere ever again. We had the greatest difficulty even coaxing her to stand, to use the toilet or be transferred from chair to wheelchair to bed, and eventually, she refused even to do that and had to be hoisted. She sat all day in a dingy corner of the lounge, installed in one of the armchairs on the pointless seat sensor, became profoundly depressed, and was dead within a year.

From pottering around town with her shopping to being wheeled out on an undertaker's gurney, all in one short year: she had us, social care, to thank for that.

There were many kinds of tears at Ember Vale: tears of rage, anger, frustration; tears of loss, grief, anguish. Tears of bewilderment. Tears of despair. Tears with no identifiable cause, welling from some unfathomable source of misery.

Some of the saddest tears were the tears of Delia for her missing children. She was mother to six, but all save one had died at birth or within their first year of life. Her surviving daughter visited as often as she could, which, as she lived on the south-west coast, was not very often, even before Covid made it impossible anyway. Most of the time, Delia recognised nobody around her and floated adrift on some far-off sea where no one could reach her. But regularly, about once a month, some fractured memories of those long-dead, long-lost children would come back to her, and she would spend hours wandering the corridors crying out for them, or sit huddled on her bed, racked by inconsolable sobs, weeping for her babies.

Perhaps because they live and work at the other end of life, carers seem almost universally to love babies and small children. When I took my firstborn to Ember Vale, he was passed round from hand to hand, and I barely saw him for a good two hours. Several of the staff who missed him that day (Lynn was one of them, annoyed that my visit coincided with her week's leave) later came to our house to coo and cuddle. When I visit my grandmother, the toddler, scurrying off, is reliably scooped up by a carer and saved from meeting a watery grave in the duckpond. Meanwhile, impeding my progress and attempts to rescue the toddler myself, an admiring crowd surrounds the baby car seat and tries to elicit smiles from the occupant within.

Ember Vale had a life-sized baby doll, and we were supposed to offer this to the residents to cuddle and care for as if it were a real baby, the idea being that this reduced agitation and aggression. Poor Delia merely took this as an insult, which seemed to me an entirely reasonable response: how can stiff, unyielding plastic compare to the warmth and softness of a living baby? How can the muteness of a doll compare to a baby's gurgles and smiles? Its stillness and lifelessness can only have reminded Delia of her baby's deaths, not of their wriggling, kicking, breathing lives.

Most of the time, the doll lay face downwards in the perambulator. Sometimes Gregory, temporarily bored of plumbing and in search of other occupation, would fish it out, hold it upside down by the legs while he took all its clothes off, and then find this hysterically funny. So the doll had its uses after all, I suppose.

My grandmother, who has always adored children, loves to have me visit with mine. She giggles at the toddler as he plays on the floor with his cars and diggers and cuddles the writhing, wriggling baby on her lap, laughing as he tries to pull her hair or touch her face. She sings to them the Austrian lullabies that she sang to my father, old, old songs he then sang to me and my siblings. When we leave, she hugs me, in tears, but she will kiss the children, and on their foreheads she will mark the sign of the cross with her thumb. This old Catholic custom always reminds me of my mother, who does the same whenever one of her children says goodbye, whether we are merely going out for the day or moving to an unknown future on the other side of the world.

One of my favourite photographs shows my grandmother, my father, my first child and me: four generations intertwined. All of us are looking at the camera except Grandma, who is looking down at the baby on my lap, wanting to have him on hers.

There is that quote from Shakespeare about old age being a return again to

...second childishness and mere oblivion
Sans eyes, sans teeth, sans taste, sans everything.

The second childhood is so much crueller than the first. Children gain independence, curiosity, energy day by day. Week by week, month by month, year by year, the world becomes larger for them. Old age works in reverse. The world shrinks and closes in again; vitality is lost; self slips away. But Shakespeare is too pessimistic. It need not be mere oblivion, sans everything. Not if there is love, and care.

7

THE BUSINESS OF DYING

Every winter a rat dies on my lawn. Always a solitary, single rat, always soggy and bedraggled, and always in the same place, so that I am half convinced it is the same rat reincarnated each year to haunt me anew. The first winter, after gazing at it for several weeks from the back bedroom window, debating whether it *was* actually a rat or merely a pile of rotten leaves, I finally went out to deal with it, armed with wellington boots, a shovel and a couple of plastic bags. Thus equipped, I advanced upon the enemy, circled it and retreated. Advanced again, and retreated again. This was repeated several times. Advance, circle, retreat. Advance, circle, retreat. Eventually, I gave myself a stern talking to: "Come on, Eleanor, pull yourself together, you can't be defeated by a dead rat." Advanced again, and gingerly, standing as far away as possible, poked the corpse with the spade. The blade sank horribly easily into the sodden matted fur, and the rat rolled over, revealing a hideously grinning mouth crammed full with long, curving teeth. The stiffened tail, longer than the body itself, twitched on the ground as if coming again to life. I recoiled. Retreated one final time in abject surrender. A dead rat had defeated me.

Now, when a fresh corpse appears on the lawn, I do not even attempt to deal with it. Instead, I holler upstairs: "David! Dead rat for you to deal with!" And, bless him, out he goes to shovel it up and inter it in the communal grave at the foot of the fence. He doesn't mind dead rats. I do. Any dead animal – be it a roadkill deer lying on the verge with legs stuck stiffly upright, a fox curled as if asleep in the hedgerow, a barely formed chick fallen from its nest – seems to provoke a physical revulsion. I can't touch them, can't look at them. Dead bodies, on the other hand, I can regard with relative equanimity. It is strange.

When I was a child, my mother had a human skull, acquired for the purposes of study during her medical student days. Occasionally, she would bring it out and show us how the separate bones fitted together, or lift off the top (it had been sawn through and fitted with a hinge) to show us how the brain would have nestled inside. The skull, who was called Albert, lived for a while under my bed (ours was a house very short on storage space), where he bothered me not at all. But one day, a friend came to visit, and we sat on the bedroom floor to play chess. In the middle of the game, she suddenly caught sight of Albert underneath the bed. She said not a word, but a most extraordinary expression came over her face. Only then did it dawn on me that it was, perhaps, not quite usual to have a skull under one's bed.

Albert aside, I was in my mid-twenties before I saw a dead body. When my grandfather died early that beautiful midsummer morning, he lay in bed until the undertakers came in the afternoon, and to his side, by primeval and spontaneous instinct, gravitated the household to hold vigil, to sit a while beside the bed, swapping stories and memories, or in quiet silence to say goodbye. It seemed entirely natural that we should do this. The unbearable tension of his dying had been released, and for a brief, suspended moment there was peace. He did not look dead, merely asleep; the cliché, it seemed, was true.

Two weeks later, I went down to the funeral parlour to 'view the body'. Midsummer was past; it was pouring with rain. I was shown first into a nondescript waiting room, as if going to the dentist. From here, a full-bosomed, brightly dressed lady – not at all my mental image of an undertaker – showed me into a tiny, windowless room at the back of the building. There was nothing in it except the coffin, barely room even for that.

I looked into the coffin. He looked the same, but he was different, in some intangible, indescribable way. He simply wasn't there. Looking down, I could feel nothing, no grief, only a terrible numbness.

I had brought with me a rose from the garden of Stonegarth, the house he had lived in for more than fifty years, the house he had died in. Reaching into the coffin, I tucked it behind the folded hands, out of sight. Beneath the hands, folded in typical pose over the breast, was a navy woollen jumper of the type he had worn day in, day out, and beneath the jumper was a terrible rigid firmness. I recoiled, not knowing why, still not knowing why, and hastened out of the room. I went back to Stonegarth, to walk the hills and woods behind the house, where he was infinitely closer to me than in that hateful little room.

That was my first experience of death close to. After this, it seemed to pick up speed. That year, in a kind of ghastly parody of the film, I went to four funerals and a wedding. Then came Covid and the care home. In those first few weeks, several residents died of or with the virus, and after that they went back to dying of what they usually died of: heart failure, respiratory failure, stroke, extreme old age. Or they simply gave up any will or desire to live, and then death, slow but inexorable, came to claim them.

Dying is a long, demanding, all-consuming job. Relatives were often surprised at how long it took, at how a frail body could cling on so long with so little sustenance. Of course there are quick deaths – a sudden, massive stroke, an overtaxed body swiftly succumbing to pneumonia or Covid or other respiratory failure – but mostly they seem to drag on, and on, and on. My mother, on my advice, for I was worried he would die before she could get there, changed her flights and came out to Stonegarth early, whereupon my grandfather hung on to life for another several weeks, finally yielding and slipping away the day before her booked return flight to Auckland. There are no guarantees in death, only that it must come.

At the care home, few relatives came to sit with their dying, even when the first barricade was lifted and this was graciously allowed again, gowned, aproned and masked, of course. Instead, it fell to us, strangers, to coax down a few drops of fluid, hold a hand, stroke a forehead. But the stillness of dying was incompatible with the mayhem of a shift. There was no time for us to help people to die well, only rush, rush, rush, and don't forget the paperwork, make sure you initial to say that you checked on room 20 and found them still dying, no familial love or proper care, only the well-meaning but clumsy administrations of strangers.

It always surprised me how many families were content to let this be. But of course no one wants to confront dying, or to look upon it; we are frightened of it, avoid it where possible, so that I started this chapter by talking about dead rats and skulls under beds, and folded the washing and put it away, and settled the children – so very young and plump and healthy – with extra solicitude before finally, reluctantly, sitting down to write about the dying of the elderly. And even now I find I don't know how to do it. It is so much easier to let dying happen behind closed doors, to come in when it is all over and look down and say, oh, Mum looks so peaceful now. But it seems to me that this deprives both sides. Families can give important, necessary, vital relief by learning to perform a few simple tasks: giving sips of water, creaming heels and pressure points, moistening parched lips, gently cleaning a dry mouth. Little things, simple things, but needing time and patience and compassion and love. And though watching someone die, especially someone you love, is utterly horrible, is there not some comfort to be had in performing these final acts of love, in knowing you did all you could? I think so. I hope so. I have found so.

Much busyness attends the business of dying. Doctors, once they have signed off the prescription for end-of-life medication, wash their hands of their patient and will never see them again – if indeed they ever did. But the district nurse will visit at least once a day, to check the syringe driver gently whirring away at the end of the bed – supposedly hidden under the sheet, but everyone knows it's there. Only the nurses have the key to unlock it; only they have the authority to check and adjust the flow of drugs; care home staff, even the manager, are not to be entrusted with this. The nurses usually come in the morning, and then throughout the day the carers will be – or should be, if only there are enough of them on shift – regularly hurrying in and out, to perform the two-hourly position changes, to change sheets and bedding, to cream elbows and heels and buttocks where the skin is breaking down, check pads, coax the taking of a little fluid and write down in the tatty OCRB – Ongoing Care Record Book – that they have done all these things. When they have, they will set the CD player going so that the dying person is inflicted with the sound of Julie Andrews or Vera Lynn or Frank Sinatra or whoever happens to be in there, and then they will hurry out and on to the next person; if they have time, they will pause a minute before they go, to stroke a hand and croon, "It's all right, Martin, all right…" Outside in the corridor there will be brief, hurried updates and exchanges, and hopefully, hovering anxiously and awkwardly on the edge of this melee, there will be the family, to whom one carer will have to be assigned to offer regular cups of tea and frequent reassurance; in spite of this, familial heads will pop out into the corridor; an anxious gaze will alight upon a passing carer; and a worried voice will ask/plead/demand/command, "Please can you come? Mum doesn't look very comfortable." No wonder most people seem to slip away in the early hours of the morning, when all is still, attendants elsewhere and family home for the night. It's the only time they can get any peace.

Studies bear this out, suggesting that many do indeed die early in the morning. Apparently, most hospital deaths occur between 3am and 4am; many care home deaths also occur in these still, silent hours. Science posits that the mechanical functions of the body are at their lowest ebb during this time; levels of adrenaline and anti-inflammatory hormones drop, which in turn can cause the airways to narrow, making breathing harder. Which makes sense. But does it not also make sense to go in the darkness, at the time so many cultures and religions say that the veil is thinnest between this world and another, unencumbered by wearisome watching, night blanketing the grief of those left behind? Who knows?

I do not know if people can choose when to die, although the numbers I know of who died alone, just when family or friends had finally left or when carers were busy elsewhere – as if waiting for this moment of privacy and seizing it when it came – makes me wonder. But I did know someone who apparently choose *not* to die. Victoria, succumbing to a chest infection at the height of Covid, sank rapidly into delirium, her breathing becoming shallow and rapid and her oxygen saturations plummeting. After three days of this, during which she had taken neither food nor fluid, the doctor, from afar, declared her to be end of life. Although he had not come out to examine her in person, all the staff – probably more used to dealing with dying patients than he – agreed. She lay on the low bed in her tiny little room, the curtain pulled against the brightness of the May day, stick thin, motionless apart from noisy, ragged breathing. No family came, although exceptions to the visiting ban were supposed to be made for those on end-of-life care, and even before this was officially, if grudgingly, approved by diktat from on high, Lynn – a good woman – would have allowed it if the family had wished, taking all the responsibility upon herself, her staff pretending not to see. But Victoria was alone that evening, barely hanging on to life, as I made her comfortable, filled out the paperwork and slipped out of the dingy room, fully expecting that in the morning she would be gone.

Morning came. I was on the early shift. Bleary-eyed, clutching mugs of tea, we straggled into the office for handover. The senior from the night shift, Ava, started the familiar litany. I was only half listening until she got to Victoria.

"Room 16... up and about."

I could not believe my ears. "Room *16*? Are you *sure*?"

"Oh yes. Been up and had breakfast and a cuppa. We were sitting with her, me and Amelia, when suddenly she sits up, bolt upright, and says, 'I'm not ready to go yet.' Gave us a hell of a shock. Thought she was a goner. But no, up she gets and walks off to the dining room. Been walking ever since."

So Victoria surprised us all, even Ava, who had an uncanny sixth sense for when people were 'going to go'. She never regained the weight she lost during her illness, and she never stopped walking, pacing the corridors day and night, dragging her quilt and blankets behind her. As far as I know – for I see her feature occasionally in photographs on the Ember Vale Facebook page – she is walking still, looking like a grey and gaunt ghost, but very much alive.

The residents were never told when one of their number died, and we were not allowed to enlighten them, which seemed to me wrong, especially where friendships had existed. Often the undertakers came very early in the morning, before the start of the morning shift, so we never saw the dead nor said a final farewell. But occasionally, when there had been a delay or someone had died later on, the undertakers would appear later in the day, always at the most inconvenient moment, which was breakfast time. One morning, as I was frantically trying to get the ten people on my upstairs corridor up and dressed and down for breakfast before the elusive hour of 9:30am, Lynn emerged from the lift, which I had called up to take down Beryl in her wheelchair.

"Put room 30 in the library," she instructed briskly. "Away from the windows."

I looked blank.

"*Undertakers*," she mouthed at me over Beryl's head.

So I had to steer poor Beryl into the library, so-called because of the pathetic little bookcase which stood there; the room was very small and windows running alongside the door looked into the corridor, also giving a view of the lift. Lynn came in behind me and fussed around with the positioning of the wheelchair so that Beryl's back was to the door and the window. And I had to wait there with Beryl while the undertakers came up with their empty gurney and took it down again with its burden. The lift was very small; the men, who were not, struggled to get the empty gurney out of the lift and struggled even more once they had loaded the body onto it. I watched through the window, trying to pretend, for Beryl's sake, that I did not know what was going on and that she did not know what was going on and that I did not know that she knew what was going on. Of course she did.

"Who is it?" she asked.

I told her.

As the gurney made its way through the home, doors were closed on residents wherever they happened to be – bedroom, dining room, lounge – so that they should not see its progress. All the staff, on the other hand, were expected to line up along each side of the front foyer. As the gurney passed, all heads bowed in a simple, silent mark of respect. Once, Jon, one of the few male staff and whom I had always thought flighty and rather shallow, crossed himself quickly, furtively, as the body passed. It was the first death he had witnessed, and I wondered if it was an expression of genuine piety or mere superstition. Nobody ever cried, but there were often damp eyes. Sometimes new staff would dissolve afterwards, and Lynn would have to comfort them in the office. But more usually, as soon as the front doors had clanged shut behind the gurney, everyone dispersed back to bedrooms, lounges, kitchen and laundry. The demands of the still-living allowed no time for the dead.

Once someone had died, their bedroom was always cleared with indecent haste ready for the next inmate. One out, one in. Usually, we packed everything up in empty boxes of incontinence pads, of which there was always an interminable supply, and handed these back to relatives at the front door. If the deceased had no next of kin, or the family did not want their belongings, they became subsumed into the general clutter of the home. Knickers were in perennially short supply, and there was always a rush to claim any going. Indecorous, yes, but care workers are nothing if not practical. Stella's books went to swell the thin ranks of the home library, which I think was only ever used by me. She had a penchant for murder mysteries and detective stories, which normally I too would have gobbled up. But somehow, I couldn't take her books home with me. I just didn't fancy them.

And then a new occupant would move in. It was always strange at first having to associate a new name and person with a room number that had previously been indelibly linked with someone else. But stranger still was the way in which all trace of a person, a life, a story, simply evaporated, leaving no sign that they had ever been there. Except, sometimes, for their knickers and books.

People like to think that their loved ones died well. They like to say, with Ophelia, *he made a good end*. But, of course, Polonius – Ophelia's father in Shakespeare's *Hamlet* – did not make a good end. He made a swift, brutal, undignified end, stabbed with a sword through an arras, having just been called a rat by Hamlet. *No shriving time allowed.*

People in care homes in Covid did not make good ends either.

Shrive is an old word for the Catholic practice of confessing one's sins and receiving forgiveness for them. When the ghost of Hamlet's father speaks of 'no shriving time allowed', he is rueing the fact that he died suddenly (murdered by his brother), without receiving the sacrament of the Last Rites and without having confessed his sins, instead heading to divine judgement 'with all his crimes broad blown, as flush as May'.

Now, whatever you may think of Catholicism – or indeed of religion generally – is it right to deprive someone of the rituals that may bring them comfort and relief at one of the most sacred times of their life, namely their death? Though you may not believe in a god, judgement, heaven nor hell, is it fair to deny others their belief, or to dismiss the importance of their belief?

Tucked away in a dingy corner of the conservatory at Ember Vale was a framed A4 copy of the 'Residents Charter of Rights' (to my pedantic annoyance, the apostrophe was missing). These rights included:

The right to privacy and dignity of care.
The right to choose when you get up and go to bed.
The right to choose your own medical practitioner and dentist and consult them in private.
The right to freely practise [more pedantic annoyance, that split infinitive] *your own religion and consult your religious leader (chaplain, priest, rabbi, pastor, imam, preacher, minister) as required.*

All very laudable, and you would expect no less, but honoured far more in the breach than in the observance (the location of the charter, barely visible, being an inauspicious start). As for access to religious leaders, well, during Covid in a care home you didn't have a snowball's chance in hell. They simply weren't allowed in. The situation in hospitals was similar. In New Zealand, a friend's mother was admitted to hospital, seriously ill, and told she was allowed one visitor, and one visitor only. So my friend had to send in the priest, not knowing if she would ever see her mother again, not allowed to say goodbye. Yet she was lucky to be allowed even this. Thousands must have died without the support of their religion and without the comfort this would have given their families.

In October 2021, the Conservative MP Sir David Amess, a Catholic, was stabbed to death during a constituency meeting. Somehow, a priest was found to administer the

Last Rites, only to be turned away by the emergency services. This caused outrage, mainly from Catholics but also from those of other religions and none. To its credit, the College of Policing swiftly updated its guidelines to facilitate access of religious leaders to crime scenes. Similar action is needed to ensure access to care homes and hospitals but, to date, none is forthcoming.

Dying in a care home is horrible and boring and terrible and tedious and also pretty predictable. In the elderly dying of old age, as opposed to some sudden major event such as heart attack or stroke, it generally follows a familiar pattern. The old and frail can go on being old and frail much longer than you might think or seems possible. But when they take to bed, having previously been, if not mobile, then at least in a routine of moving between bed and chair – or when an already sparrow-like appetite becomes drastically diminished – these can be signs that the end might be beginning.

It can be difficult to pinpoint when someone starts actively dying, but there is no mistaking once they are. More and more time is spent drowsy or asleep. Confusion worsens. Many wander back to childhood and earliest memories, talking to Mother and Father, or slipping out of English to another, first-learned, tongue. Less and less is eaten, as difficulties with swallowing increase. Meals will be blended up into mush, then replaced by jelly, ice cream, custard – anything soft and easier to swallow – and these too will come to be refused. Less and less is drunk, and what is coaxed down is spluttered back up again. The lips dry out and the tongue becomes furry; the mouth turns black, to be cleaned gently with a soft baby toothbrush; older carers will sometimes dip the brush in pineapple juice to loosen the thickening saliva, although due to its high acidity, this is no longer recommended. If not already present, incontinence sets in. Despite regular position changes, pressure sores can form on the buttocks, hips, elbows, heels or lower back. These are usually seen as a sign of neglect, but even with prompt, sustained care and attention – so hard to give in the melee of ever-changing shifts – they are very difficult to prevent in bed-bound patients with skin thinner than rice paper. Once established, they are even more difficult to heal. *Skin breaking down* was a familiar entry in the OCRB books, and we would slather on the Cavilon – a barrier cream prescribed to almost all the residents yet, like incontinence pads and knickers, always in short supply. Some of the seniors afforded this the reverence due to a mythical magical potion, but the cream nevertheless did very little to heal pressure sores, and too often the district nurses would have to be called out. But there was little they could do either except apply dressings that always fell off and berate Lynn for neglect, who in turn would berate us and exclaim, in capital letters every time, that we MUST DO BETTER OR RISK FAILING AN INSPECTION. POSITION CHANGES EVERY TWO HOURS AND MAKE SURE YOU RECORD IT. And so the great twin gods of documentation and action planning would be satiated, and much good this did the poor person with pressure sores.

Most of the dying were prescribed end-of-life drugs, usually midazolam for delirium or agitation and morphine, or another opioid, for pain. They were not always used, but the prescriptions would be collected from the pharmacy in readiness. I disliked doing this, feeling that I was holding death in my hands – unreasonably, since the responsibility for administering them was, of course, not mine. But it was even worse when the drugs should have been administered and were not. I remember Edith screaming out as we tried, as gently as possible, to turn her and change her pad. Every movement and every touch called forth a terrible, primal cry of pain. I forget now whether the drugs had not been prescribed or whether the nurse had just not been out to administer them, but, shocked and distressed, we went to Lynn and begged her to do something.

The drugs – thankfully, Edith did eventually get morphine for pain relief – were delivered subcutaneously through a syringe driver. Once this was set up, death usually followed within about twenty-four hours (my grandfather's carers were astonished that he hung on for nearly a week after the driver was installed). A great calmness would settle upon the dying person, a strange and stark contrast to the crying, shouting, screaming and thrashing that often went before, and the room would become very still.

They say that hearing is the last sense to fail. There is a soundtrack to dying – the gentle hum or whir of the syringe driver, the occasional groan of the airflow mattress, stirring to life in a vain, last-gasp attempt to prevent those dreadful pressure sores. (The latter can be uncanny and more than once caused me to jump like a startled cat.) If you are lucky, you will be spared the soundtrack of Julie Andrews or Frank Sinatra and perhaps have classical music instead, or perhaps just the sound of the curtains gently rustling at the open window. The noise of feet tramping up and down the corridor, even the relentless, incessant noise of the call bells, recedes; even we felt this, closeted with the dying. Sometimes the call bells can wait.

What used to be called the death rattle – noisy, laboured breathing as the patient struggles against accumulating secretions in the airways – is not actually a sign of imminent death, though people often take it to be, as it looks and sounds so alarming. The really-close-to-dying are very quiet, very still – so quiet and still that you have to stop, look and listen to discover that life is, in fact, still there. How often I have done this – and how often, now, I do it at the other end of life, looking anxiously down on my deeply sleeping babies, consumed with the terrible, irrational, yet universal fear, known to all mothers, that their child has stopped breathing in its sleep.

Many of the residents did finally stop breathing in their sleep, in those still, dark hours of the early morning. The night staff would wash and dress them and lay them out on the bed, ready for the undertaker. Usually, they were gone by the start of the morning shift, but if not, we were allowed to go in one by one and say goodbye, or otherwise pay respect. Almost everyone did. There was little fear of dead bodies; what went before was so often worse. The front door closed behind the undertakers, and our duty was, at last, discharged.

Perhaps I have made all this sound too matter-of-fact and uncaring. Of course the deaths upset me, but, like everyone else, I had a job to do and no choice but to get on with it. Collapsing in a puddle of tears and emotion would have been of no help at all, to anyone. In contrast to the NHS, pouring money and resources into its mental health days and Well-being Wednesdays and guidance and counselling and debriefing and talking therapy, there was no support for us except what we could give each other. We had to get on with it. So we did.

Sometimes it did all get too much; when Beryl was dying, the girl assigned to her corridor, who was very new and very young, simply couldn't cope. Nursing the dying is always difficult, not only emotionally but also physically. Beryl's weight and size made turning and changing her almost impossible. There were no other care staff free, so Lynn quietly stepped in (the only thing she ever did quietly) and, with Amelia, nursed Beryl herself until she died at 11am that morning. Then, when the undertakers had been, she sat with the girl in the office, arm round her in defiance of the social distancing rules, allowing the phone to ring off the hook, ignored. She looked after us all as best she could, residents and staff. It was not her fault that the care all round so often fell short.

I don't like talking about things that have deeply affected me; not for me a graphic discussion of 'birthing stories', which so many other women seem to go in for, even the normally non-garrulous. I just want to forget the whole thing as quickly as possible. Nor do I willingly talk about the care home and what I witnessed there. Writing is different; it is cathartic, and there are things I want to put on record (*not* my 'birthing stories') so that they are not forgotten. But there are things I find I cannot write about, cannot be matter of fact about. There are memories too painful, seared too deep. One of these goes back to when my grandfather was dying, to one evening so difficult to witness that it was years before I spoke of it to anyone. I thought I could write of it here, but now it comes to it, I find I cannot.

And yet, I am glad I was there.

8

NIGHT SHIFT

Most of the staff at Ember Vale worked either nights or days; only a few did both, in a routine that must have played havoc with their body clocks. Semi-mythical creatures of the night, casually breezing in at 9pm with immaculate make-up when the rest of us were hot, dishevelled and longing for a drink or a fag, or both, the night staff rather looked down on the day staff as having it easy. Perhaps we did. The workload at night was considerably and undeniably lighter, but then you had to stay up all night.

Night staff never worked days; in fact, they were often treated as privileged beings, probably because they were so hard to find. Most people, unsurprisingly, don't want to work nights. But the day staff were often drafted in to cover night shifts when, inevitably, they were short staffed. So I did a few and heartily disliked them. Working at night obviously suits some people – though they are a rare breed – either because they have children to care for during the day, or because they are naturally night owls. I am not a night owl. I like to be asleep by 10pm at the latest and sleep through until at least 6am. By far the hardest part of early motherhood for me is the relentless sleep deprivation; it induces a kind of madness. Incidentally, I wonder if this is partly why rates of dementia are higher in women than men; some dementia research suggests that lack of sleep increases risk, and it is of course women who are, generally, the ones to be up night after night, sometimes for years. A cheery thought, when the baby wakes at 10pm, and 12am, and 2am, and 5am, again and again and again, until you want to scream at them to *just sleep, please please please*!

Given that the night shifts started at about the time I generally start thinking about going to bed, I wondered rather apprehensively how I would cope. Would I even be able to stay awake all night? In the event, I had no trouble staying awake, primarily out of necessity but also because care homes, with their bright corridor lights and their infuriating bells, are not conducive to sleep, even for their residents. For the first couple of hours, I was even relatively bright and perky, but around 11pm, a kind of bone-deep fatigue descended like a cloud, and the rest of the shift would pass in a strange, dreamlike state of exhaustion and mental fogginess that felt as if it would never end. A bit like early motherhood, really.

It is a strange feeling, working while the rest of the country sleeps. But while Britain is asleep, the other side of the world is awake. I would walk up and down the corridors wondering what was happening at home, thinking of my parents and siblings going off to work and university, shops and supermarket, doing all the normal everyday things I once did too in the harsh, clear light of the Antipodes, light that is like nowhere else in the world. And the fluorescent light in the ceiling corridor, black-spotted with dead flies, would flicker and go out and come on again and flicker miserably on and off for the rest of the night, for it was perpetually broken and the electricians who appeared at regular intervals never managed to fix it for long.

"Cleaning. Lots of cleaning."

Lorraine had said this in answer to my question as to what night shifts were like. I had to ask her twice, because she was night staff and therefore superior to the day staff and, when eventually she deigned to notice me, had given this laconic reply.

There was indeed a lot of cleaning. During the day, domestics were employed, separately from the care staff, but at night all the cleaning had to be done all over again by the carers. We had to clean all the toilets and bathrooms, all the lounges, wet mop the dining room and foyer and vacuum all the corridors. My mother used to say that cleaning toilets is very grounding. That's one way of looking at it.

The cleaning was punctuated by the hourly rounds to check on each resident in their room, always called 'doing the bells' or just 'the bells' because we had to press the mute button on each call bell in each room. This would register with the system and prove that someone had indeed been in to check on the resident at regular intervals throughout the night. Some of the night staff could whip in and out so quickly that they could barely have noticed whether the occupant was alive or dead. But it was documented on the system, which was all that mattered.

Cleaning done, there was laundry to tackle. Again, a laundry assistant was employed during the day, but only by having the carers put loads on overnight could she hope to keep even remotely on top of the mountains that had to be done. (I feel for Hannah. I can barely keep on top of the washing for my own family of four. But I used to envy her, working calmly away in the laundry room or ironing by the open window, soundproofed from the call bells by the gentle white noise of the two huge washing machines and two equally huge dryers.) Laundry baskets stood on every corridor and were always overflowing by the end of the day. No attempt was made at sorting beyond separating soiled (with blood, vomit, urine or faeces) from non-soiled. Soiled washing went into red plastic bags, or green ones if the fabric was delicate; these bags went straight into the washing machine on their own extra hot wash and, by some magic that none of us could quite fathom, dissolved completely in the wash. All the washing, dark and light together, was hastily hurled into the machines – industrial-sized and so large that a smallish adult could have curled up inside – in a slapdash manner that would have horrified my mother and mother-in-law. (The highest compliment the latter ever paid me was to approve of my washing technique, though I'm not sure I quite live up to my mother's.) Slam went the door, in went the washing powder into detergent drawers caked with years-old powder half an inch thick, and that was another job done. On to the next.

"Did you see Ruby?" Sheryl asked after my first night shift.

I was confused. The home had no resident, nor member of staff, named Ruby.

Ruby, it transpired, was a previous resident, now the resident ghost. Apparently, she liked on occasion to hang out in the kitchen and dining room, where she would indulge in a spot of mild haunting during night shifts – lights turning on and off, doors opening of their own accord, that kind of thing. Why her hauntings were restricted to the dining areas nobody seemed to know. Perhaps, like the members of the family I had married into, she was ruled by her stomach.

Care workers are the most practical and down-to-earth people I have ever met, but at the same time, many seem to combine this with a certain superstition. Perhaps it is inevitable, working at the interface between life and death. As for me, I do happen to believe in ghosts, but I never saw Ruby. I don't think I would have been scared of her, but I'm glad I didn't know about her before that first night shift.

I never saw Ruby, nor have I ever seen any other ghost, but – as in many lives – things have happened that perhaps could be explained rationally, or perhaps not. As I drove home after that first night shift, through a world still sleeping although already bathed in the warmth and light of a fine summer day, I was thinking of my grandfather. It was the anniversary of his death two years before, when the sun had risen to just such a morning. As usual, I had the car radio on, and as I turned into the road where David's parents lived, a piece began whose crashing opening notes I recognised immediately. It was Sibelius's *Finlandia*, written in 1899 as an assertion of Finland's independence against the overweening power of neighbouring Russia. It was music loved by my grandfather, and I always associated it with him. It was played at his funeral; I had spent hours beforehand cutting the nine-minute piece into two smaller sections, to be played through my laptop as the coffin was carried into the church for the service and afterwards out again for the last time. I had overestimated how long it would take for the pall-bearers to reach the altar – it was only a small church – and the music had played on long after they had reached it and placed the coffin on the trestles, echoing and reverberating around the rafters as the small handful of black-clad mourners stood in silence below.

I turned the car onto the driveway and switched off the engine, but the radio played on, and I sat there, in front of the still-sleeping house, listening, alone in a world of music and sunlight and memory. From that dramatic opening, the piece gives way to a slow and solemn march, gathering force into mounting darkness and menace; then suddenly the tone changes to a light and joyful dance which slows to quietness and rest, before building again to the final triumph and passion and defiance. When it ended, I turned the radio off and sat there for a long time.

It was not so surprising that the piece should have been played. As anyone who listens regularly to Classic FM will know, they have a rather limited repertoire, and pieces are repeated with what sometimes feels like a distinct lack of imagination. So I hear *Finlandia* occasionally, although not as often as, say, Bruch's Violin Concerto No. 1, or anything from Karl Jenkins' *The Armed Man*, which in my humble opinion is played far too often. (I like the Bruch.) But was it beyond coincidence that it should have been played that early morning, just a few hours after the time my grandfather died, after a night spent in the watchful darkness, closeted with those on the edge of life, some of them about to cross the great, unbridgeable divide? Who can tell? Does it matter? It was odd and unexpected, but I took comfort from the music and a sense that death need not shut out those we love. And I went into the house, just as everyone else was beginning to wake up, went to bed and tried, unsuccessfully, to sleep until lunchtime.

In spite of Ruby's possible presence, the dining room was where the night staff congregated to sit out the darkness and wait for dawn. After cleaning and laundry, unless someone died, there were long hours between about 2am and 5am, punctuated only by the bells. We would assemble at one of the tables with the books and, assisted by tea and toast, sit down to smash out the paperwork. This would never have been tolerated during the day, but discipline was much laxer at night, and in many respects the night staff were a law unto themselves. Often, they worked out of uniform, wearing only a singlet, claiming that the building, always hot and stuffy, was infinitely more so at night. Tunics would be casually thrown on again a couple of minutes before 7am as the day staff, at this point still semi-fresh and ironed, began to congregate in the office for handover. This was flagrant breach of the regulations, but the night staff would remain aloof, sallying homeward almost as immaculately made up as when they floated in, fortified by that tea and toast and a nice little mid-shift sit-down, unwearied by the constant harried hoisting, lifting, pushing and rolling which characterised the day shift.

Doing the books was much quicker at night. The entries ran along the lines of *So-and-so had a quiet night*, or, at most, *So-and-so had a quiet night. Pad change 2am.* So they were swiftly dealt with, and once out of the way, there was time for talk. And another cup of tea. The night shifts had fewer staff than days: a senior and just two carers, one of whom was responsible for the 'upstairs' residents and the other for the 'downstairs'. This meant that the night team was very tight-knit, partly because it was small, partly because there were long hours with little to do but talk. The night staff knew every detail of each other's lives, every member of each other's families. Often their lives intertwined outside of work as well as within it. I, who always at Ember Vale felt an outsider, could only sit on the fringes of these conversations, where I was usually ignored anyway, and would sit curled up in a stupor of exhaustion which cup after cup of weak tea could not fend off. It was always a relief when the first faint chirpings of the birds outside heralded the dawn. The other two would languidly rise and stretch; tea mugs were returned to the kitchen; and off we went to 'start getting people up'.

Care home residents go to bed early, often aided by lorazepam, typically prescribed for anxiety or sleeplessness. In fact, the night staff were quite put out if there were more than three or four people still up when they came on shift. People are so much less trouble once they are tidily tucked away in bed asleep. But it is not right. Yet another case of infantilising the elderly, yet another mockery made of the 'person-centred approach'.

One recent evening just after 7pm, and just after putting to bed my four-month-old baby and nineteen-month-old toddler, I rang another care home, where my grandmother had been placed for a period of respite care following a fall which had fractured her hip. Usually, care home phones ring and ring and ring because everyone is too busy to answer them. This one was picked up with surprising alacrity.

"Hello-please-can-I-speak-to-Mrs-Bloomfield?" I said in my best telephone voice, über-polite and slightly too rushed.

"No, you can't," said a bald, bored voice at the other end. "She's in bed."

"But she isn't usually in bed at this time!" I said.

If a voice can be said to shrug, this one did. "Well, she's in bed now. And I ain't going down to get her up."

I was gobsmacked. I ought not to have been, of course; I knew how care homes work. It's just that, apparently, you don't expect them to work like that to your own.

They go to bed early, and get up early. It's the only way to get through everybody, to get everyone through the dining room by that arbitrarily appointed hour of 9:30am. At Ember Vale, the night staff would start getting people up around 5am. They always started with Florence, that tiny ball of white fluffy hair and hissing invective and latent coiled energy. She would snarl, scratch and spit her way through washing and dressing, then – once tucked up in her armchair beneath a blanket to which she would cling for dear life – promptly fall asleep again until her porridge was dumped in front of her three or four hours later. Depending on how hard the night staff felt like working, after Florence they would either get up seven or eight more or a mere two or three. If the latter, the morning staff would groan and look daggers, for it meant they would be behind all day. It shouldn't be like that, of course it shouldn't, but the rights of the individual are subordinate to the demands of the institution. That's how it works, that's the only way it can work, and unless or until care homes are properly staffed, that's the only way it will work.

I still do a night shift, but it's at home now, fashioned around the whims of babies who fail to recognise that their mother would be a better mother if she had some decent sleep. Up at night with her own children, my sister-in-law thinks of me, or of the other mothers all over the world, an exhausted, wakeful army, soldiering on through the darkness. But I think of the care home and the hot, still hours of the night, of the bells and the rounds, of the suffering that is temporarily muted by sleep, of the souls that may slip away during those strange, unworldly hours. And when I do manage to fall asleep, perchance to dream, my dreams take one of two themes; it has been that way since 2020 when the world changed. One is of home, New Zealand, where it is always summer, and the sea is always somewhere nearby. The other, more nightmarish, from which I am always glad to wake but which always leaves a lingering residue throughout the day, is of the care home.

9

THE DARK SIDE

It takes a lot to faze a care worker. Blood, puke, wee, poop, life, death – they have dealt with it all. They work early, late and through the night, weekday, weekend and holiday without discrimination. They are paid a pittance and receive little, if any, thanks. They are given little training of any practical use and no support. They see things that cannot be unseen, hear things that cannot be unheard. They worked unlauded and unrecognised through a two-year pandemic. They try – mostly – to help the lost and lonely, to ease suffering, to care. And they do it day in and day out. Until they don't. For care work breaks everyone in the end.

In this I speak of those employed in care work – not those who do it unpaid for a relative or, less usually, friend. In familial situations, love, affection and duty owed can call out superhuman feats of strength and endurance, perhaps as necessary compensation for the additional anguish and guilt imposed. But for those whose job is care, these bonds, and therefore these compensations, do not hold. Care work is often hailed as 'not just a job'. True: it is all-consuming. It takes over your life and erodes the boundaries between work and home. It dictates family life and has a detrimental effect on relationships. And it will chew you up and spit you out without a second thought.

Of those I worked with at Ember Vale, maybe three or four are still there. Otherwise, the little tribe of people with whom I worked for a time has scattered like pollen on the wind. A few moved on to more prestigious roles, usually hospital-based, within the NHS. Several disappeared all at once, during the cost-of-living crisis in the winter of 2022, when soaring costs meant they could no longer put fuel in the car or afford the bus fare to work. Most commonly, after simmering unhappily for weeks or months, people finally reached the point when the hours, the pay (or lack of it) and the stress became overpowering. Then they quit abruptly, often without working out their notice or finding another job, simply walking out of the front door and never coming back.

And one was sacked, or, in employment-speak, 'lost her position'.

This episode was deeply troubling. It was badly handled; we were told nothing and forbidden to discuss it, expected to carry on as if nothing had happened. Of course everyone did discuss it, furtively in the corridors in hushed tones, always looking over one shoulder in case Lynn or someone from head office should suddenly heave into view. The atmosphere in which we worked, never exactly pleasant to begin with, became unbearably tainted. Trust vanished. Everyone was suspicious of everyone else. People suddenly became obsessed with documentation and witnessing to the point of paranoia.

It began one busy lunchtime when one of the girls – I'll call her Shirley – suddenly left the building in floods of tears after being closeted with Lynn in the manager's office. This was annoying – we were now one staff member down at one of the busiest times of the day – but not necessarily unusual. Shirley suffered from severe migraines and did sometimes have to leave a shift because of them. I continued doling out plates of stringy roast beef swimming in watery gravy and thought no more of it.

Lunch over, busy moving people out of the dining room and into the lounge, I passed Grace taking down some of the profile photographs from the staff board in the foyer. This seemed a bit odd, but plenty of things at Ember Vale were a bit odd, and as Grace would not have graced an enquiry with a reply, I did not bother to investigate. Passing the main office, I saw through the glass of the door that one of the residents – I'll call them Lindsay – was sitting inside. The door was closed, and the sign had been moved to the red 'engaged', which meant that we were not allowed to enter. This too was a bit odd, as it was not the doctor's day (if the resident was not bed-bound, consultations always took place in the office, weekly on a Friday at the changeover of shifts when we all needed to get in the office to complete timesheets, check rotas and hand over notes). But again, not necessarily unusual.

Back in the lounge, two carers were huddled together in one of the darkest corners, discussing something in hushed tones. Something in their manner made me go over and ask: "What's up?"

A confused story emerged. Lindsay had been found to have bruising on their upper arms, marks consistent with being pulled upwards from a seated position by somebody standing in front of them. Asked how these had been sustained, they had said, "One of the girls." Lindsay had been showered the previous evening and Lynn assumed, for no particularly clear reason as far as I could see, that the bruises had been inflicted then. Shirley had given the shower but categorically denied assisting Lindsay to stand in a non-approved manner or causing any bruising. Faced with this denial, Lynn had given orders that Lindsay should be shown the photographs of the staff members working the previous shift and asked to pick out the 'girl'.

I had worked the previous shift. Now distinctly alarmed, I went to look at the photo board again. My photograph was among those missing.

I felt a sickening lurch of fear. The elderly, with their paper-thin skin, bruise easily; it can happen even when moved according to correct handling techniques. Like everyone, I worked always in a hurry, always hoping that nothing amiss would happen, always torn between the resident I was assisting at the time and the other three or four all clamouring for my attention too. What if I had been careless, unforgivably rushed, and caused the bruising? Lindsay disliked me, I knew that; they apparently disliked everyone but reserved especial disdain for me. What if, motivated by malice, they picked my photo out of the line up? Then again, Lindsay had poor eyesight and some level of mental incapacity. What if they picked my photo by mistake, or on a whim? I would lose my job, instantly, dismissed without a reference. Marking a resident, whether accidentally or not, was the cardinal, unforgivable sin from which there was no redemption.

I did not lose my job. Shirley did. Lindsay picked her photograph, and she was suspended pending an investigation whose result was a foregone conclusion.

I did not believe, and still do not, that Shirley deliberately caused those marks. Perhaps she was unwise. Perhaps, struggling to help Lindsay to stand by pushing from behind at the waist, having them try and fail to brace against a slippery wet room floor, to save time she went round to the front and, against the regulations, pulled them up and forward, rather than calling for help she knew would not come. Or perhaps she did nothing wrong, and the marks were caused by another person, another time. Unwise or innocent, she was a good carer. Yet all her years of service and experience, all the accumulated good she had done – all were blotted out in a moment. Nobody stood up for her. We had worked alongside her, liked her, respected her work. But everyone was preoccupied with their own position, knowing that the same thing could easily have happened to any one of us. Shirley was one of us; we could so easily have been her. Rather than admit this, the entire home, as if by silent, communal agreement, never spoke of her again. She vanished like a stone dropped in the ocean, leaving as little trace. Lynn had forbidden all mention of her and any attempt to contact her, but she did not need to. The carers self-censored, and Shirley was completely ostracised.

This bothered me so much that eventually, after much private deliberation, I defied Lynn's injunction and messaged Shirley on Facebook. The message was along the lines of *Hey, hope you're doing OK, thinking of you, let me know if there's anything I can do.* I saw that the message had been read, but never received a reply.

Work was different after Shirley's departure. People were warier, more cautious. Many would work only with their particular friends. Like others, I started refusing to work alone with difficult residents without a witness. In a world that did nothing to protect us, we tried to protect ourselves. In some ways, I think Shirley was a scapegoat, dismissed to make an example of and to strike fear into those left behind; the company could hardly have sacked everyone for every accident and shortcoming, or they would have had no staff left. But always now we had one eye over our shoulder, worried in case 'something should happen'. So, when something did happen, and it was my name that was given in to Lynn for investigation, I was very worried indeed.

Let's call this resident Their Royal Highness, which is how the carers referred to them. Nothing was ever quite right for Their Royal Highness, who would do nothing for themselves even though they had full mental capacity and, compared to most of the residents, pretty good physical capacity as well. They complained incessantly about everything. Most of these complaints were not worth bothering about, but one night they complained that they had lost £100 in cash. More specifically, that it had been taken from their bag. More specifically still, that the carer who had been assisting them that night must have taken it. That carer was me.

It is a horrible feeling, being falsely accused of theft. The police were called and turned up, looking very bored, the next morning. They interviewed Their Royal Highness, full of weepy righteous indignation, in the office, while I hovered in the corridors outside trying to be busy, sick with suspense. They did not formally interview me, but I was asked to write a statement:

I was assisting TRH with evening personal care... they asked me to pass them their bag as they wanted some money from it. I did so... they looked in the bag and said £100 was missing... they became very upset and wanted me to help them look for it... we looked together in the bag and then TRH asked me to search the room... I did so but could not find any money. TRH became even more upset, and I said I would have to report this to the senior... I went to find the senior who came back with me to talk to TRH... TRH said that they had lost £100 and that I must have taken it because I was the only person who had been near them all evening... the senior and I searched the bag and the room again but did not find any money...

The money, if it ever existed, was never found. In general, residents were not allowed to keep cash on their persons or in their bedrooms for precisely this reason, the risk of it going missing. If a resident wanted cash (none ever did, for they had little opportunity of spending it), it was withdrawn for them and then locked in the office safe. No cash was listed on the inventory of TRH's personal possessions made, as was standard practice, when they entered the home. No money had been withdrawn for them by care home staff. The family, when asked, had not done so either. So the matter was allowed to drop, although not before I had spent a very sleepless night. If it came down to a carer's word against a resident's, the business of Shirley had left nobody in any doubt that it would be the resident's which was heard. But nothing more was done, except that all the care staff were told not to deal with Their Royal Highness unless there was a witness present. The police constables, looking more bored than ever, took my statement – handwritten, in rather shaky writing, with a failing Biro on sheets of printer paper – and let themselves out. It probably languishes to this day in some forgotten police file.

In between chivvying and browbeating her staff, sacking some and calling the police on others, Lynn tried to maintain some semblance of morale, a thankless and largely impossible task. Nobody, staff or residents, harboured any illusions about Ember Vale; an exhausted cynicism reigned supreme. If you survived, you were doing well. Nobody thrived.

As part of this brave but doomed attempt to keep up morale, and also keep up appearances via photographs on Facebook – *look, here are our lovely carers being recognised for their hard work while residents* [mostly asleep and almost without exception unaware of what was going on] *look on and applaud* – awards ceremonies were held every quarter, which we were all expected to attend whether on shift or not. NG would occasionally turn up at these to preen and simper and take any credit that was going. The company nominally sponsored these awards, but the idea was Lynn's. Poor Lynn, they never really got off the ground. Everyone came dragging their feet, resenting either coming in on their days off or being forced to take time from work that needed to be done. But they really became a dead duck when it transpired that the extra three hours' annual leave awarded to those who had maintained a 100% attendance record over the quarter could not be used. The company claimed some technicality, I forget what, but there was outrage, outrage which was, as usual, entirely impotent.

Why did I stay? Why didn't I leave, like the others? All the time I worked at Ember Vale, I was looking, looking for other jobs. To this day, a graveyard of over a hundred rejected job applications sits on my computer hard drive. Nothing came of any of them. And so, since our mortgage depended on my employment, I had to stay.

How did I stay? I had been brought up not to give up, to grit your teeth and keep going. I had stubbornness in abundance, and pride. So I gritted my teeth behind my mask and kept going. But it got harder and harder, and at home, outbursts of angry, bitter tears became more and more common.

Late one night, when we were still living with David's parents, I came home utterly exhausted and boiling over with rage. I forget now what had triggered the simmering tension and tipped me over the edge, but it was midwinter, not long after my miscarriage. I had cried bitterly for the baby that would never be, but also felt a secret shameful disappointment that there would be no break for maternity leave as I had expected, that I was still stuck at Ember Vale. Something, probably something very minor, must have happened at work to make me snap, but I remember only standing at the bottom of the stairs, lacking the energy or the will to climb them, and the storm of tears, a great deluge of accumulated futility and helplessness, humiliation and horror. I remember, too, the look on David's face: wordless, frozen shock. I remember the guilt of making him look like that.

I said, or rather sobbed, that I could not go back, would not go back. I meant it.

But – the mortgage.

And so, the next morning, without anything being said about the histrionics of the night before, I went back.

But that night I sat up late, gin to hand, scribbling furiously in the notebook that I had previously used for my PhD work, words tumbling out in a foaming, boiling torrent. In time, those words became this book.

When eventually I did leave Ember Vale, it was, ironically enough, by walking out of the front door and never going back. But I did not know it at the time, and it was not my decision.

Another baby appeared. This one decided to stick around. Covid restrictions on hospitals and midwife appointments being still in full force, it was not a particularly pleasant time to have a baby. But one of the restrictions worked to my advantage. Official government advice apparently stated that pregnant women in their third trimester should not be working in frontline healthcare roles. In practice, this caused endless confusion. The care company said it was the midwife's decision to state whether or not I was fit to work. The midwife said it was the care company's responsibility to ensure they complied with government advice. After going round in circles for several weeks, I gave up and simply sat back to see what would happen.

Lynn, as usual, was in a quandary. She could not afford to lose a worker. Equally, she could not afford to be in breach of official regulations. Eventually, she came up with a compromise: she would transfer me to the receptionist's role, currently vacant, so that I worked in administration rather than on the care rota. She put this forward to head office for approval on the day that I went off for two weeks' summer leave.

I spent the leave looking for nice beaches in Devon to remind me of home, and praying fervently that head office would accept Lynn's proposal. No doubt the receptionist's role came with its own stresses and pressures, but they seemed preferable to those of working on care. The hours were set, a civilised 8:30am–4:30pm Monday to Friday; no early mornings, late nights or weekends. No seniors demanding to know why the dining room wasn't cleared yet. No toileting. No back-breaking lifting, hoisting, rolling or pushing. No wrestling Florence through the shower. A lot of telephone and computer work, liaising with the incoming medical professionals, dealing with residents' family and friends. In comparison to care work, it seemed a doddle. All right, dealing with Georgina's daughter wasn't a doddle, but I had to do that anyway. I'd take the daughter if it meant getting off care.

After a week, I heard back from Lynn. Apparently, the guidance stated that from the third trimester, pregnant women should not be working in healthcare settings at all, whether or not they dealt directly with patients or, in the case of care homes, residents. I was to be signed off on medical leave with immediate effect. It was the first, last, and only time that I was grateful to Covid regulations.

So I never went back from my summer leave. As for maternity leave, I spent it outwardly vowing that I would not go back and inwardly terrified that I would be forced into going back. There were bills. And the mortgage. And saving up to go home, should the New Zealand border ever reopen. But, less than two months before I was due back, I applied for a job in the university library. This time, finally, I got it.

I was lucky. Very, very lucky. Make no mistake: if it were not for that break, I too would eventually have snapped completely. Everything would finally have got too much: the misery, the pettiness, the bells, the smells, the paperwork, the handover messages pinging relentlessly through three times a day, the endless pleas for cover, the dreams, the nightmares. I would have walked out of that front door, not to two weeks' leave, but to no alternative job and no reference.

And Lynn, that ever-smiling, irrepressible bundle of sturdy resilience? Everything eventually got to her too. I heard on the grapevine, shortly after my first baby was born, that she had suddenly and unexpectedly resigned with immediate effect. She too walked out of that front door and never came back.

The meanness of the company apparently knew no bounds. One teabag per shift – the cheapest possible, PG Tips, bought by the thousand – that was what we were allowed. We had to pay for every part of our uniforms, our DBS checks, even the key fob that some preferred to use in order to let themselves into the building rather than wait up to fifteen minutes for someone to be free to answer the door. If you were a fraction late for a shift, your pay was docked accordingly. If you had to leave a shift early, because of illness or emergency, your pay was docked accordingly. There was no pay for being forced to come in every Wednesday to complete a postal PCR Covid test, even if you were not rostered to work that day. (We found ways round this. Initially we took kits home to complete and post on the Wednesday morning; then, when they cottoned on to that and started counting the number of kits out of the care home, making sure they tallied with the number of staff, we simply completed them on an earlier shift and left them in the pile to be collected on Wednesdays.) There was a continuous and predictable cycle regarding the leftover food from the residents' dinners and teas: this was not supposed to be eaten by the carers, but, having served the residents, everybody would take a bit here and there to eat over their breaks. Every so often, there would be an angry missive from head office saying that we had to pay for this; then a few weeks later, there would be an even angrier missive saying that leftovers had to be thrown out rather than given to staff; then, gradually, everybody would slip back into quietly appropriating a sandwich here or half a baked potato there. Some of the seniors would shamelessly pile up a plate until it overflowed, then retire to the office to consume their spoils. (The food was not very good. The same dishes were served over and over again; fresh fruit was practically unheard of, as was fresh juice; tea was sandwiches, crisps and dinner's leftover pudding, day in, day out; and everything was overcooked to a soft mush. But you get hungry on a physically active seven-hour shift. And no, Georgina's daughter, the food was not organic.) The taking of leave was strictly controlled: it could be taken only in week blocks, Monday to Monday; you could take a maximum of two weeks back to back and a maximum of two weeks in any quarter; you had to work the weekend before your leave started and the weekend after your return. We had to buy necessary items of clothing or toiletries for residents upfront, then be reimbursed a month later, rather than being given the money out of the office petty cash; when you live pay cheque to pay cheque on a very meagre wage, this is not always easy. No, there were no perks at Ember Vale; the meanness was all technically legitimate and within the company's rights, but petty in the extreme. They could not even stand us a drink at Christmas time. Lynn did, out of her own pocket.

The company clearly did not grasp the basic premise that if you look after your employees and treat them with a modicum of respect, they will be happier, more loyal, more hard-working and less likely to leave. Or, more likely, they simply did not care. So everyone was intensely unhappy; nobody had a shred of loyalty to the company or the home; nobody felt inclined to go above and beyond the call of duty; and everybody got the hell out of there whenever the opportunity presented itself.

Of course, the real losers in all of this were the residents, who could not leave and had no autonomy over their own lives. They had the most basic necessities of life: food, warmth, shelter. But not the most necessary thing of all: love. Most of the staff tried, most of the time, to give care and compassion, respect and dignity. But often, so often, we fell short, foiled by the pressures of time or the weaknesses of human nature: frustration, impatience, quick-temperedness, apathy, sullenness. Carers are not angels. They are human, with human faults and failings, too often exacerbated by the conditions they work under. At the height of the pandemic, there was a sudden spike of media coverage focusing on NHS nurses, medics and healthcare workers experiencing 'compassion fatigue'; in the years since, various academic papers have been published on this topic. The definition of compassion fatigue can be broad and nebulous but usually includes the concept that those caring for others, especially under emergency conditions, reach a state of such physical and emotional exhaustion that they have nothing left to give. It becomes too hard to care, so you simply stop caring. Under this definition, the entire staff of Ember Vale, if they stayed long enough, reached this point. It's nice to be able to put an academically recognised label on it. But academic labels don't help the residents.

Residents became lost amid the regulations and procedures supposedly there to protect them. Individual character was forced to be subordinate to the institutional whole, a whole much less than the sum of its parts: all those individual stories lost, personalities dulled, reduced to choosing between faggots or fish on Friday lunchtimes. Nobody ever truly settled at Ember Vale. Most, if not all, were admitted against their will, as Lynn, ever honest, freely admitted. Once ushered kicking and screaming – whether metaphorically or literally – over the fateful threshold, all deteriorated rapidly, both mentally and physically. During the first month or so, we mopped up endless tears and fielded endless distraught questions: why am I here? Why did my family put me here? When can I go home? Then, the first storm over, most stabilised into a horrible state of depression and drastically reduced mobility. From there many died very quickly, usually within the year. A few – like Martin, he who simply starved himself to death – deliberately gave up and went within the month. The rest hung on in the shadows, some with a degree of resignation, some trying to the last to get out. Julian, every evening, would pack up his pitifully few clothes, books and photographs – firstly into his suitcase and then, when that was taken off him, into a Tesco bag he somehow scrounged from somewhere. Then he would go and sit in the foyer, waiting for the taxi that would take him home. Every morning the carers would unpack his bag, and every evening he would pack it anew.

10

CARING FOR YOUR 'LOVED ONES'

This was written on the sign above the front door, in fancy italic script: *Ember Vale. Caring for your 'loved ones'*. The ironic quotation marks, presumably inserted either by someone with a less than adequate grasp of English grammar and punctuation or someone with an extremely fine sense of dramatic irony, always seemed to me entirely appropriate. If you truly loved your loved ones, you wouldn't put them in Ember Vale.

About forty staff worked at Ember Vale, and not one of them, from the kitchen assistant to Lynn herself, would have willingly put a family member into residential care. There you have the clearest possible indictment of the country's care home system.

And yet many people who find themselves in a position of responsibility for an elderly relative turn to care homes as if to a saviour. Some see a care home as the only option. Often, it's not. In-home care is kinder and more effective and a lot more can be done at home than many people realise. (But please don't be cross with your carers if they turn up late to a home visit because, as with residential care, they will be working under impossible time pressures.) Some people – a minority, I want to think and believe, but they do exist – see elderly relatives as a burden to be rid of and a care home as a convenient answer. Several residents at Ember Vale, despite having family members living close to hand, never received any visitors at all, nor even so much as a phone call. Carers are not much given to heartbreak, but this was genuinely heartbreaking, and in corridors or staff room no attempt was made to conceal the contempt felt for these absent family members. Carers judge families. They know instinctively who cares and who doesn't, and it will be mentally noted down and never forgotten.

Most families have no idea what a care home is really like, even if they do visit regularly. Partly this is because – of course – the home puts its best foot forward when family are around. But the family also don't want to know, because the reality is too hard to face and compounds guilt. When families move a relative into residential care, they often offer the excuse, 'it's time to hand over to the professionals'. But what they don't, or won't, realise is that care home staff are not professionals. Those at the lowest end of the pay scale, and therefore the people who actually do the caring rather than the paperwork, are people like me: completely untrained and unqualified, largely unsupported, working in terrible conditions, probably a danger both to themselves and the people they care for. A few will be excellent carers despite everything, and the majority will leave at the first opportunity. Can you be sure that it is the former who is looking after your loved ones and not the latter? Given the laws of probability, is it likely?

Disputes over care can tear families apart, adding another level of pain and grief to an already intensely stressful situation. This happened to my father's side; the family is fractured and splintered, fractious and fraught, which led to a comical reunion scene at the Royal Infirmary, where in spite of being intensely anxious to avoid each other most of us somehow managed to converge on the same hot and sticky afternoon. The poor ward staff had to deal not only with a diminutive but determined eighty-eight-year-old Austrian hell bent on absconding but also with a coterie of tense, anxious, irritable relations, most desperate to avoid talking to each other. Comical on one level – but on another, so deeply, deeply sad.

My mother's father died at home, after a prolonged and heroic effort to keep him there, necessitating various changes to the layout of the house and, gradually, more and more external help. My father's mother was able to stay at home for a lot longer than most people thought possible but eventually fell in town and fractured her hip, leading to a ten-day stay in hospital and then a period of residential respite care. Despite the best efforts of Camp Keep At Home to get her back there, it was eventually ruled impossible; she would have required twenty-four-hour live-in care, not permitted under the terms of the sheltered accommodation where she had been living. The move to the care home became permanent.

So, I have seen care both at home and in a home, and have experienced care homes both from within (as a staff member) and without (as a family member). For what it's worth, this is my two pence.

Quality of life at home is undoubtedly superior to that in a care home. Much can be done at home to help a person continue to live there as long as possible. Hoists and chairlifts can be installed. A bathroom can be converted into a wet room. Most crucially, external help – carers, physiotherapists, speech and language therapists, podiatrists, district nurses – can be put in place, and the level of help, the bulk of which will come from the carers, can be increased as necessary. Yes, this is expensive, but so is a care home; average fees are around £800 per week. Most are much more than this. And the vast majority of residents really, really hate care homes. They hate being locked in. They hate being cut off from family, friends and the outside world – for they are cut off, whether by visiting hours, the fact that the telephone line doesn't reach the ends of the building (Ember Vale), the fact that the phone isn't cordless so can't be carried to a resident (my grandmother's care home), the fact that the television signal can't be persuaded to work in the bedrooms (pretty much any care home anywhere), or simply the fact that a partially blind, partially deaf ninety-two-year-old isn't very good at Facetiming. They hate being attended to by an ever-changing rota of staff who call them darlin', babe, or a mispronounced diminutive of their first name.

If a care assessment concludes that someone shouldn't be in a care home but at home, then home is where they should be. But if, having done all you can, you absolutely must put someone you love in a care home, then please listen when people who know try to tell you what it's really like. Forewarned is forearmed. Don't make the mistake of telling yourself that the care home you have found is different from all the rest. They are all pretty much the same. Make a nuisance of yourself: speak to the manger, the assistant manager, the receptionist, the seniors, the activities coordinator, the kitchen staff, but most of all, make sure you speak to the carers. These are the people who will be looking after your loved one at the most intimate level on a daily basis, and they are the ones who won't be introduced to you when you visit to look round, because they will be far too busy trying to care for people. Demand to speak to them. Ask them how long they have worked there and what their short- to mid-term career plans are. Ask them what they find most challenging about working there, and most rewarding. Ask if they mind you asking what they get paid, because a company that pays its carers only minimum wage doesn't care about them and, by extension, doesn't care about your 'loved ones' either.

Once you have chosen a home and moved your loved one in, visit as often as you can. When you can't visit, telephone. With Covid now behind us, you should be able to visit at any time of day or night, although in practice homes often restrict visiting hours; families are a nuisance and get in the way of the smooth running of the home. Persist. Ask to be involved in your loved one's care – something practical like giving a bath or shower once a week. Check the wardrobe and drawers every now and then; clear out the rubbish that will inevitably accumulate there and make sure they have enough clothes, especially knickers or underwear, always the first items to go missing. Take your loved one on trips out of the home as often as you can. If they can't go far, at least get out into the garden, if there is one. If they are wheelchair-bound, consider providing their own personal wheelchair rather than relying on the care home's inevitably inadequate fleet of antiquated and grubby machines. Don't wear a mask to speak to the elderly; they won't be able to hear you and the distance created is acutely distressing. Decorate your relative's room, bring in as many pictures and photographs as you can, so that the carers can gain a sense of who your relative is and who their relatives are. Put a pot plant in the room and bring in flowers. In the midst of death and dinginess, both carers and residents like to look at something fresh and living. Ask to see the care notes, medication notes and food and fluid charts. Keep talking to the carers and try to develop a working relationship with them. Learn their names. Thank them, and mean it. When the time comes, ask to be part of the end-of-life care.

The building I now work in, part of the university library, is the old county asylum. The former wards and cells have been converted into open-plan office space and meeting rooms of various sizes. Anodyne spaces, now, all scrupulously clean, well ventilated, carpeted in a discreet, institutional grey. But the building is Grade II listed and so many of its original features have been preserved, if you know where to look for them. Many of the windows – not on the frontage but tucked away down the side wing – are still barred, to prevent escapes. The glass window panes in one of the big office spaces has scratchings etched into the glass – the graffiti of former inmates, nearly two centuries old. The stone walls of the turret staircase seem to be particularly thick, and there is a room on this staircase – once a caretaker's guardroom, now one of the smallest meeting rooms – that always chills me whenever I enter it. Step inside, and the gentle hum of the library beyond dies away; in the cool dimness of this little stone-walled room, there seems to linger only a great sense of sadness and suffering and loss.

As understanding of mental health conditions, and the ability to treat them, improved, asylums became a byword for places of cruelty and mistreatment. Now, though, the pendulum is subtly swinging back the other way. Without attempting to deny or downplay their myriad problems, there is a gradually dawning awareness of the shades of grey. Nothing is ever black and white. A new narrative is emerging that, although terrible, unforgivable things did occur, and great unhappiness was rife, this was not deliberately sought or intended. The university archive includes a comprehensive document, seventy pages long, outlining the rules for the management of the asylum – a sort of nineteenth-century charter of residents' rights. But asylums, especially as the resident populations increased, were overcrowded and understaffed. The staff that did exist were often untrained and unsupported, with no idea how to handle challenging and sometimes violent behaviours. They cared, but they couldn't cope.

I sometimes wonder if the popular narrative around care homes will, in time, follow a similar trajectory. When people wake up to what really goes on in them and how they are really run, will there be an outpouring of outrage and condemnation? Will there be demand for change: more staff, more qualified staff, better training, improved treatment of employees, greater respect all round for both residents and staff? Will the outrage and condemnation, in time, then give way to a recognition that, by and large, the overworked and under-resourced staff have, for years, done the best they can under extremely challenging conditions?

For that is the thing about care workers. They fall short again and again and again, and they know it. No one knows it better than they. But, in spite of everything, they do the work that no one else wants to do, again and again and again. Someone has to do it.

AFTERWORD

Everyone says to me now that I have landed my dream job. I work in the archive of the university library, with rare books and manuscripts and boxes and boxes of archival material dealing with history, literature, culture, science and sometimes the downright bizarre. I fall down fascinating rabbit holes looking for answers to researchers' queries. There are no call bells; the reading room is a beautiful haven of scholarly quiet. (It is also freezing cold. That is my only complaint.) I read lots, write a bit (mostly answers to enquiries, but also for outreach), struggle with my rusty German translating some of the letters held in the archive. I teach a very little bit – just enough to keep my hand in, not enough to dislike it. I curate exhibitions based on material held in the archive – work new to me, but I enjoy it. I learn and have the chance to learn. It is work I am good at, and I am very happy there.

So yes, I have landed my dream job. But it was a long and bumpy road to get there. Although I have been at the university for more than a year now, I still cannot quite believe I made it back into academia. It feels odd now to work in an environment where the most urgent problem is which researcher's enquiry to deal with first; where taking a break is actively encouraged; where the whole team can make time together for tea and cake in the office; where, if I do not finish what I am working on by the end of the day, I can leave it until the next without causing harm or negligence. I am still astonished at my good fortune and still so very, very grateful.

I was not good at care work. I tried, but I was too inexperienced, too untrained, too unsupported, too temperamentally unsuited to the stress, the pressure, the relentlessness, the noise. I hated working at Ember Vale. I hated that I hated it, working so closely with people who were so vulnerable and so alone. I should have helped them, but I could barely help myself. I failed those I cared for in so many ways: compassion, understanding, time and, yes, care. It was not all my fault; much of it was the fault of the system and the circumstances. But I still feel guilty.

So, this book is for the residents – an apology.

And it is for the carers – an offering.

In 2022, as the turbulent waters of Covid started to recede, the entire NHS was awarded the George Cross, in recognition of its seven decades of service and the efforts of its workers throughout the pandemic. The George Cross is the highest order of civilian award, given for 'acts of the greatest heroism or of the most courage in circumstances of extreme danger'. My sister-in-law, who is an NHS speech and language therapist, spent a year working from home, seeing children remotely via video call; when the therapists were finally allowed back into face-to-face clinics, they had to work with the children at a distance of two metres while wearing full PPE, including masks (makes speech work difficult, that). So she is aware of the irony of having a George Cross for courage, and has mislaid her lapel pin.

Meanwhile, the contribution of carers and care staff goes unmarked. Towards the end of 2020, NG issued all the staff at Ember Vale with a cheap, tacky enamel lapel pin; it had *CARE* written in white lettering across a plain green background. We were supposed to wear them pinned onto our tunics. Only Lucy, always obedient, ever did.

When my grandfather died, his coffin was carried by his two sons, his son-in-law, his stepson, one of his grandsons – and one of his carers. My mother and grandmother, trying to work out the funeral arrangements, could initially only think of five pall-bearers.

"What about Will?" I said.

They had not thought of him. But they asked him, and he said yes. It seemed to me entirely appropriate that, having provided so many thousand acts of personal service, he should also perform this final one, one last time.

After the funeral and the burial, we went back to the house for the wake. The food and drink was laid out in the dining room, which was the room where he had died; it had been turned into a bedroom when he could no longer make it up the stairs, even on the chairlift. The dining table and chairs, which had seen so many family dinners down the years, had been sold a few months prior to make room for the hospital bed. Most people took their food from the sideboard and made their way to eat in the lounge, but a few of us stayed in the dining room, perching on the two remaining antique armchairs, leaning against the bay window, or sitting on the floor. A lot of alcohol was drunk and the freely flowing wine seemed to heighten clarity rather than diminish it. I noticed hundreds of tiny golden hairs from the rug – I was sitting on the floor, just where the bed had been – sticking to my black tights. They would not brush off.

Will and Rachel, the two carers, were talking about their work. They worked in community rather than residential care, but much of what they said was to become so familiar to me, less than two years later. The hours. The pay. Company bureaucracy. The gruelling physicality of the work. The lack of time to care properly. Management who did not understand what care work actually entailed.

But they also spoke with warmth, wit and compassion about what should be the centre of care: the people. They saw so much suffering, but amid the drudgery and the anguish, they relished the idiosyncrasies, the personalities and, yes, the vitality of their patients. If you don't laugh, you'll cry. They chose to laugh.

"I remember this time," Will was saying, "we was running late for a client, a couple, and we hurried up the stairs two at a time, and in we burst on them, *doing it*. And I remember thinking, bloody hell, man, you're both in your eighties, neither of you can get out of bed on your own, but you're still doing it! I mean, good on you. If you got it, you got it. Good on them."

I am a wordsmith, trained in words, to interrogate and inspect them, to wield them with precision and force. So I went and looked up the etymology of *care* in the Oxford English Dictionary.

Care, noun: from the Old English *caru, cearu*: mental suffering, sorrow, grief, trouble. Serious or grave mental attention; the charging of the mind with anything; concern; heed, heedfulness, attention, regard; caution, pains.

Care, verb: from the Old English *carian, cearian*: to sorrow or grieve. To be troubled, uneasy or anxious. To feel concern, be concerned, trouble oneself, feel interest.

To care for: to take thought for, provide for, look after, take care of.

That sums it up, I think.